Register Now for Online Access to Your Book!

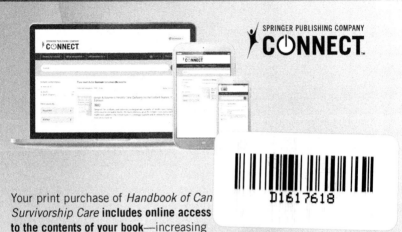

SPRINGER PUBLISHING COMPANY
C NNECT.

D1617618

Your print purchase of *Handbook of Can Survivorship Care* **includes online access to the contents of your book**—increasing accessibility, portability, and searchability!

Access today at:
http://connect.springerpub.com/ content/book/978-0-8261-3825-5 or scan the QR code at the right with your smartphone and enter the access code below.

Scan here for quick access.

0SG6J4KG

RC271.M4 H36 2018
08006335
Handbook of cancer survivorship care /

The online access with your
is available at the publisher'
may be removed at any time

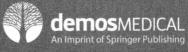

demosMEDICAL
An Imprint of Springer Publishing

View all our products at springerpub.com

SPC

Handbook of Cancer Survivorship Care

Editors

Maria Alma Rodriguez, MD
Professor, Lymphoma/Myeloma
Vice-President, Medical Affairs
Office of Chief Medical Officer
The University of Texas MD Anderson Cancer Center
Houston, Texas

Lewis E. Foxhall, MD
Professor, Clinical Cancer Prevention
Vice President, Health Policy
Office of Chief Medical Officer
The University of Texas MD Anderson Cancer Center
Houston, Texas

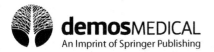

demosMEDICAL
An Imprint of Springer Publishing

Visit our website at www.springerpub.com

ISBN: 9780826138194
ebook ISBN: 9780826138255

Acquisitions Editor: David D'Addona
Compositor: diacriTech

For Figures 10.1, 10.2, 10.3, 11.1, 11.2, 12.1, 13.1, 14.1, 14.2, 16.1, and 16.3, the cancer survivorship algorithms have been specifically developed for MD Anderson using a multidisciplinary approach and taking into consideration circumstances particular to MD Anderson, including the following: MD Anderson's specific patient population; MD Anderson's services and structure; and MD Anderson's clinical information. These algorithms are provided as informational purposes only and are not intended to replace the independent medical or professional judgment of physicians or other healthcare providers. Moreover, the algorithms should not be used to treat pregnant women.

Medicine is an ever-changing science. Research and clinical experience are continually expanding our knowledge, in particular our understanding of proper treatment and drug therapy. The authors, editors, and publisher have made every effort to ensure that all information in this book is in accordance with the state of knowledge at the time of production of the book. Nevertheless, the authors, editors, and publisher are not responsible for errors or omissions or for any consequences from application of the information in this book and make no warranty, expressed or implied, with respect to the contents of the publication. Every reader should examine carefully the package inserts accompanying each drug and should carefully check whether the dosage schedules mentioned therein or the contraindications stated by the manufacturer differ from the statements made in this book. Such examination is particularly important with drugs that are either rarely used or have been newly released on the market.

Library of Congress Cataloging-in-Publication Data
Names: Rodriguez, Maria Alma, editor. | Foxhall, Lewis E., editor.
Title: Handbook of cancer survivorship care / Maria Alma Rodriguez, Lewis E.
  Foxhall, editors.
Other titles: Cancer survivorship care
Description: New York : Springer Publishing Company, [2018] | Includes
  bibliographical references and index.
Identifiers: LCCN 2018013749 | ISBN 9780826138194 (alk. paper) | ISBN
  9780826138255 (ebook)
Subjects: | MESH: Cancer Survivors—psychology | Survivorship |
  Neoplasms—psychology | Neoplasms—therapy
Classification: LCC RC271.M4 | NLM QZ 260 | DDC 616.99/40651—dc23
LC record available at https://lccn.loc.gov/2018013749

Printed in the United States of America.
18 19 20 21 22 / 5 4 3 2 1

Contents

Contributors

Maria Suarez Almazor, MD, PhD   Professor, General Internal Medicine, The University of Texas MD Anderson Cancer Center, Houston, Texas

Amin Alousi, MD   Associate Professor, Stem Cell Transplantation, The University of Texas MD Anderson Cancer Center, Houston, Texas

Joann L. Ater, MD   Professor, Pediatrics, The University of Texas MD Anderson Cancer Center, Houston, Texas

Spyridon Basourakos, MD   Genitourinary Medical Oncology, The University of Texas MD Anderson Cancer Center, Houston, Texas

Therese Bevers, MD   Professor, Clinical Cancer Prevention, The University of Texas MD Anderson Cancer Center, Houston, Texas

George J. Chang, MD, MS   Professor, Surgical Oncology, Professor, Health Services Research, The University of Texas MD Anderson Cancer Center, Houston, Texas

Alejandro Chaoul, PhD   Assistant Professor, Integrative Medicine Program, Department of Palliative, Rehabilitation, and Integrative Medicine, The University of Texas MD Anderson Cancer Center, Houston, Texas

Lorenzo Cohen, PhD   Professor, Integrative Medicine Program, Department of Palliative, Rehabilitation, and Integrative Medicine, The University of Texas MD Anderson Cancer Center, Houston, Texas

Joyce E. Dains, DrPH, JD, RN, FNP-BC, FNAP, FAANP   Professor, Department of Nursing, The University of Texas MD Anderson Cancer Center, Houston, Texas

Suzanne Day, MSN, RN, FNP, APRN   Cancer Prevention Center, The University of Texas MD Anderson Cancer Center, Houston, Texas

Beatrice J. Edwards, MD, MPH   Associate Professor, General Internal Medicine, The University of Texas MD Anderson Cancer Center, Houston, Texas

M. Kay Garcia, DrPH, LAc   Associate Professor, Integrative Medicine Program, Department of Palliative, Rehabilitation, and Integrative Medicine, The University of Texas MD Anderson Cancer Center, Houston, Texas

Katherine R. Gilmore, MPH   Project Consultant, Office of Cancer Survivorship, The University of Texas MD Anderson Cancer Center, Houston, Texas

Alison Gulbis, PharmD   Stem Cell Transplantation and Cellular Therapy, The University of Texas MD Anderson Cancer Center, Houston, Texas

Jeri Kim, MD   Genitourinary Medical Oncology, The University of Texas MD Anderson Cancer Center, Houston, Texas

Marita Lazzaro, MSN, RN, ANP-BC, APRN   Cancer Prevention Center, The University of Texas MD Anderson Cancer Center, Houston, Texas

Paula Lewis-Patterson, DNP, MSN, RN, NEA-BC   Executive Director, Office of Cancer Survivorship, The University of Texas MD Anderson Cancer Center, Houston, Texas

Wenli Liu, MD   Associate Professor, Integrative Medicine Program, Department of Palliative, Rehabilitation, and Integrative Medicine, The University of Texas MD Anderson Cancer Center, Houston, Texas

Gabriel Lopez, MD   Assistant Professor, Integrative Medicine Program, The University of Texas MD Anderson Cancer Center, Houston, Texas

Haleigh Mistry, MS PA-C   Lymphoma/Myeloma, The University of Texas MD Anderson Cancer Center, Houston, Texas

Ellen Mullen, PhD, APRN, GNP-C   Lymphoma/Myeloma, The University of Texas MD Anderson Cancer Center, Houston, Texas

Tilu Ninan, RN, ANP-C   Cancer Prevention Center, The University of Texas MD Anderson Cancer Center, Houston, Texas

Jeong Hoon Oh, MD, MPH, FACP   Associate Professor, General Internal Medicine, The University of Texas MD Anderson Cancer Center, Houston, Texas

William Osai, MSN, NP-C   Genitourinary Medical Oncology, The University of Texas MD Anderson Cancer Center, Houston, Texas

Guadalupe R. Palos, DrPH   Manager, Clinical Protocol Administration, Office of Cancer Survivorship, The University of Texas MD Anderson Cancer Center, Houston, Texas

Linda Pang, MD   Assistant Professor, General Internal Medicine, The University of Texas MD Anderson Cancer Center, Houston, Texas

Kristen B. Pytynia, MD, MPH   Associate Professor, Head and Neck Surgery, The University of Texas MD Anderson Cancer Center, Houston, Texas

Maria Alma Rodriguez, MD   Professor, Lymphoma/Myeloma, The University of Texas MD Anderson Cancer Center, Houston, Texas

Johnny L. Rollins, MSN, APRN, ANP-C   Manager, Advanced Practice Provider, Department of Endocrine Neoplasia and Hormonal Disorders, The University of Texas MD Anderson Cancer Center, Houston, Texas

Charles Schreiner IV, MHA, MS, RN, ACNP-BC, APRN   Head and Neck Surgery, The University of Texas MD Anderson Cancer Center, Houston, Texas

Karen Stepan, MPH, RN, MCHES   Program Manager, Psychosocial Oncology, The University of Texas MD Anderson Cancer Center, Houston, Texas

Karen Stolar, MS, FNP-BC, AOCN   Stem Cell Transplantation, The University of Texas MD Anderson Cancer Center, Houston, Texas

Lynn Waldmann, LCSW   Sr. Social Work Counselor, The University of Texas MD Anderson Cancer Center, Houston, Texas

Angela Yarbrough, MSN, RN, FNP-BC   Pediatrics, The University of Texas MD Anderson Cancer Center, Houston, Texas

Preface

Survivorship is now recognized as a critical and separate phase of the cancer care continuum (1). The Institute of Medicine (IOM) report, *Lost in Transition*, increased awareness that coordinated follow-up care can enhance the overall health and quality of life for cancer survivors (2). Since the IOM report, notable advances have been made in the care of survivors who have completed curative treatment, including development of clinical algorithms and guidelines, emergence of survivorship care plans, progress in health policy initiatives, and increase in clinical education for healthcare professionals caring for cancer survivors. The IOM report identified four domains as core concepts in providing comprehensive care to survivors. They included surveillance for new/recurrent cancers, management of late or long-term effects, risk reduction/prevention, and monitoring psychosocial functioning.

To address the growing needs of cancer survivors, in 2008 the Cancer Survivorship Program at MD Anderson Cancer Center launched a robust clinical program that provided tailored care designed for long-term cancer survivors. In response to the various advances and changes in survivorship care and the desire to provide high-quality survivorship care, the Cancer Survivorship Program added educational and research components. In 2018, there are 12 different disease-specific survivorship clinics delivering care to adult survivors of the most common cancers such as breast, prostate, colorectal, and gynecological cancers. However, clinics have been added for other cancers, including thyroid, head and neck, lymphoma, and our most unique stem cell transplants. The clinics were and continue to be based on a multidisciplinary model of survivorship care, which includes the principles set forth in the seminal IOM report. These core elements are embedded in our institutional clinical care program, practice algorithms, and survivorship care plans. These domains serve as the foundation for the delivery of multidisciplinary care for survivors.

In our experience, one notable gap continues to contribute to the unmet needs of cancer survivors—the limited availability of educational resources for healthcare professionals, particularly those in primary care, which focus on this unique population. To provide coordinated care and appropriate care plans, practitioners must have educational resources that focus on the complex and unique management of cancer survivors. Despite the widespread recognition of their value, there are few, if any, published handbooks to educate practitioners about the complex nuances of survivorship care.

Clinical handbooks covering the basics of survivorship care are one way to provide up-to-date strategies to the oncology workforce, that is, oncologists and other primary care providers. Such resources must be concise, user-friendly, and easy to access for practitioners in diverse and busy clinical settings. *Handbook of Cancer Survivorship Care* addresses, in detail, the current and practical management of long-term cancer survivors. The content in this handbook is written in a manner that can be easily applied in a variety of clinical settings and practices.

CONTENT

This text consists of 16 chapters that are organized into two sections. The handbook serves as a practical and useful guide for the multidisciplinary management of long-term cancer survivors.

Part I: General Principles of Survivorship Care covers basic principles of survivorship that aid the clinician in the assessment and management of survivors' care. The goal of this section is to help establish the foundation for content covered in Part II. Chapters 1 and 2 introduce the reader to core concepts of survivorship; provide a review of the IOM's core domains; and present a definition of cancer survivorship and long-term cancer survivors. Chapter 3 provides a detailed discussion of the basic concepts of surveillance, late effects, and prevention of new or secondary cancers. Chapter 4 outlines the psychologic challenges that often accompany the survivorship experience. Strategies for cancer screening and prevention are discussed in Chapter 5, with application to the needs of long-term cancer survivors. Chapters 6 and 7 focus on the complex care of older survivors, older than or equal to 65 years, and provide a useful discussion of late effects and comorbid conditions that create a confluence of special needs for this population.

Part II: Management of Site-Specific Cancers contains everything needed by clinicians to provide quality care to cancer survivors. Chapter 8 discusses the role of integrative medicine in addressing some of the late effects of cancer and its treatment. The handbook is designed for care of the adult survivors; however, Chapter 9 addresses the burdens faced by adolescents and young adults who are survivors of cancer. This section also focuses on cancers selected by the editors because they were the sites with the largest number of survivors seen in the clinics or are considered the most common in long-term survivors. Readers will discover that Chapters 10 to 16 in Part II offer guidance on surveillance, prevention, late effects, and psychosocial issues encountered by cancer survivors. The outline format provides evidence-based, easy-to-use information that can be integrated at the point of care regardless of clinical setting or specialty. The handbook features a concise overview of a specific type of cancer with a discussion of the clinical tools, that is, survivorship algorithms available for the practitioner.

Nearly all the chapters are written by a team working in a survivorship clinic, including a seasoned oncologist who specializes in the specific cancer disease and an experienced practitioner who provides direct patient services. By using a team approach, we combine the clinical expertise of experienced practitioners with an expert oncologist who has a broader understanding of the theory and research of that particular cancer.

Brief clinical vignettes illustrate the application of the clinical practice algorithm(s) and survivorship care plan developed for each type of cancer. An outline format gives the reader concise and easy access to the survivorship guidelines and other information to support their application.

We believe this practical, concise, and easy-to-read handbook will become the go-to book on cancer survivorship for practitioners in diverse clinical settings. Each chapter will contain useful and state-of-the-art information on the application of clinical algorithms and personalization of survivorship care plans for specific subgroups of survivors. The handbook's size and availability of the ebook format will also increase its appeal to trainees, oncologists, and other providers.

AUDIENCE

Handbook of Cancer Survivorship Care is a practical and useful resource for a widely diverse number of audiences within the spectrum of oncology, primary care, family medicine, nursing, and other important specialties. There are other groups who will also benefit from this clinical handbook. The first are hospitals or academic centers who offer training programs to residents, fellows, or other trainees in various subspecialties. The second are practitioners in community-based hospitals caring for cancer survivors who have returned to their local communities for follow-up care. The third are academic institutions preparing the future oncology workforce. This market group includes schools of medicine, nursing, osteopathy, pharmacy, and other similar academic institutions.

Maria Alma Rodriguez and Lewis E. Foxhall

REFERENCES

1. Zapka JG, Taplin SH, Solberg LI, et al. A framework for improving the quality of cancer care: the case of breast and cervical cancer screening. *Cancer Epidemiol Biomarkers Prev*. 2003;12(1):4–13.
2. Hewitt M, Greenfield S, Stovall E. *From Cancer Patient to Cancer Survivor: Lost in Transition*. Washington, DC: National Academies Press; 2006.

Acknowledgments

The editors would like to acknowledge Demos Medical Publishing, whose support and patience guided the production of this clinical handbook. We also wish to acknowledge the work of Brenda Feinberg, whose expertise in medical editing contributed significantly to the quality and completion of this textbook, and to Kathy Carpenter for her diligence in keeping track of all the deadlines associated with the production of this book. We also appreciate the work of Ubong Atiata, Jacqueline Gonzales-Carmona, and Natalie Suarez, the college trainees selected for the Survivorship Research Internship who worked "behind the scenes" on several logistical, operational, and technological aspects of the book. Finally, and most important, we thank our contributing authors for their expertise, time, and commitment to making this clinical handbook a one of a kind.

General Principles of
Survivorship Care

Defining Cancer Survivorship

Maria Alma Rodriguez
Paula Lewis-Patterson

CANCER SURVIVOR DEFINITION

The Institute of Medicine's (IOM; now the National Academy of Medicine) landmark report, *From Cancer Patient to Cancer Survivor: Lost in Translation*, raised awareness of the need to address the specific issues that cancer survivors encounter after completing their cancer treatment (1). In 1986, the National Coalition for Cancer Survivorship introduced one of the first definitions of *cancer survivor* by stating that a patient who has had cancer is a cancer survivor from the time of diagnosis through the remainder of his or her life (2). This broad definition takes into account the entire spectrum of the cancer journey—diagnosis, treatment, remission, surveillance, after-cancer care, and end of life. The cancer journey affects caregivers, family members, and friends; therefore, all of these people also are recognized as survivors. The National Cancer Institute (NCI) customized the definition of survivorship, stating that it is the "health and life of a person with cancer post treatment until the end of life" (3). Survivorship encompasses the physical, psychosocial, and economic issues of cancer beyond the diagnosis and treatment phases. Survivorship involves issues related to the ability to obtain healthcare and follow-up treatment, late effects of treatment, second cancers, and quality of life (3). The focus of this chapter is the care of adult survivors who have completed their curative treatment. This handbook's authors acknowledge NCI's definition and recognize survivorship as a distinct period that commences after treatment is complete and the time during which recurrence most likely has passed. Healthcare providers in all types of clinical settings and practices need to prepare to care for growing numbers of cancer survivors.

This chapter introduces basic concepts used in the specialty of cancer survivorship such as risk stratification and survivorship care models that transition survivors from treating oncologists to providers who specialize in survivorship care. A clinical vignette demonstrates how survivorship concepts, models, and risk stratification can be integrated into routine clinical practice.

SURVIVORSHIP STATISTICS

According to statistics from the Surveillance, Epidemiology, and End Results (SEER) database, approximately 15.5 million cancer survivors resided in the United States in 2016 (4,5). SEER data estimate this number will increase to 20.3 million by 2026.

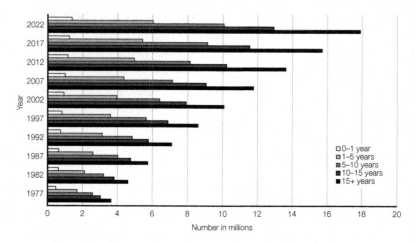

FIGURE 1.1 Cancer survivor statistics by age group.
Source: Adapted from de Moor JS, Mariotto AB, Parry C, et al. Cancer survivors in the United States: prevalence across the survivorship trajectory and implications for care. *Cancer Epidemiol Biomarkers Prev.* 2013;22(4):561–570. doi:10.1158/1055-9965.EPI-12-1356

By age distribution, 74% are 60 years of age and older, 21% are 40 to 59 years old, 4% are 20 to 39 years old, and fewer than 1% are younger than 20 years old (4,5). Approximately two-thirds of patients with cancer live at least 5 years after receiving their diagnosis, with many survivors living 15 years or longer after diagnosis (Figure 1.1). The most common cancers for men are prostate, colon, rectum, and melanoma, whereas breast, uterine corpus, and colorectal cancers are the most common cancers for women (6).

FORCES DRIVING SURVIVORSHIP CARE

In 1985, Fitzhugh Mullan, a physician and cancer survivor, published "Seasons of Survival: Reflections of a Physician with Cancer" (7). This article chronicled his personal cancer story and launched a movement in which patients with cancer shared their concerns related to life after cancer treatment (7). Dr. Mullan's work and the IOM report gave cancer patients a forum in which to voice their concerns regarding the impact of symptom management (physical and psychosocial) after treatment, the onset of late effects, and poor coordination of medical care attributed to a lack of communication among providers (1,7). Other factors contributing to the increase in cancer survivors include an aging population, early detection, and improved treatment modalities (8).

In 2013, the IOM published a second report, *Delivering High-Quality Cancer Care: Charting a New Course for a System in Crisis,* which called for a dramatic shift in the broken, cost-prohibitive cancer-care delivery system. This care model defined survivorship as a distinct cancer care phase (9) and described a patient-centered, evidence-based approach to care; a system for sharing of critical patient information; and ways to cultivate collaborative practice among all caregivers. Organizations such as the Centers for Disease Control and Prevention, NCI, and the American Cancer Society continue to highlight the need to recognize and address cancer survivors' long-term needs. The Commission on Cancer, an accrediting body, has published quality measures focused on improving cancer care (10). The measures mandate that an all-inclusive treatment summary and follow-up plan be provided to patients who complete curative cancer treatment. Chapter 2 provides a detailed description of these critical documents and their role in survivorship care.

DOMAINS OF SURVIVORSHIP CARE

The premise of survivorship care is to shift patient care from a model of illness to one of wellness. Typically, patients are transitioned to a survivorship clinic after surviving beyond the interval during which risk is highest for recurrence of their primary malignancy. The IOM outlined four domains for the delivery of survivorship care: surveillance, monitoring for late effects, preventive services, and psychosocial health (1). These domains are listed in Figure 1.2.

Cancer surveillance and screening

- Detection and treatment of late malignancy recurrence or new second malignancies

Late effects/side effects management

- Health maintenance and observation of vital organ function

Risk reduction and cancer prevention

- Lifestyle changes to prevent cancer and risk assessment

Psychosocial functioning

- Psychosocial support services to maintain healthy relationships and restored life

FIGURE 1.2 Core domains of survivorship care as recommended by the Institute of Medicine.
Source: Institute of Medicine. *From Cancer Patient to Cancer Survivor—Lost in Transition: An American Society of Clinical Oncology and Institute of Medicine symposium.* Washington, DC: The National Academies Press; 2006.

Surveillance is conducted to detect recurrence of the primary malignancy and assess for the likelihood of any second cancer. Prevention counseling is provided to encourage lifestyle changes including but not limited to smoking cessation, healthy living, energy balance, and dietary changes. The body of knowledge regarding the late effects of cancer treatments comes predominantly from studies of childhood cancer survivors. Children who received anthracycline during treatment and are now in their 40s and 50s are experiencing accelerated coronary artery disease (11–13). The body of knowledge regarding late treatment effects for adults with cancer continues to grow.

Other cancer-treatment modalities such as radiation may increase risk for other symptoms and conditions (11). Therefore, screening for late effects based on the specific treatment received is essential. The psychosocial and economic consequences of surviving cancer treatments are as important as the physical late effects. Patients and their families often face many challenges, including economic stress, loss or disruptions of relationships, and emotional distress that may last or manifest long after therapy is completed.

SURVIVORSHIP CLINIC MODELS

The University of Texas MD Anderson Cancer Center has three types of survivorship clinics that can serve as models of care for cancer survivors:

1. In the first model of care, survivorship patients transition from their primary disease treatment site to a cancer prevention center with multidisciplinary healthcare providers. Clinical leaders in cancer prevention provide operational oversight of these clinics. Included in this model are patients with breast, thyroid, and colon cancers.
2. A second model is one in which disease-specific clinics, such as genitourinary, melanoma, and sarcoma clinics, provide survivorship care within each of their each disease-specific centers. A steering committee with representation from each primary oncology discipline (radiation, surgical, and medical) within the center governs the operation of each clinic. The primary oncology discipline refers patients to clinics in which care is delivered based on the four domains of survivorship care.
3. A third model is referred to as a comanagement model and is used in MD Anderson's hematology malignancy clinics. Patients who have received a stem-cell transplant schedule visits with a survivorship provider when they see their stem-cell transplant physician. Clinical operations are governed through an internal operations leadership team.

THE INTERDISCIPLINARY SURVIVORSHIP TEAM

The emergence of survivorship as a distinct phase of cancer care carries with it established and new knowledge regarding care delivery, practice, and technology. To address these issues, MD Anderson has developed survivorship practice algorithms. Each disease-specific algorithm defines patient eligibility, surveillance, late effects, risk reduction and prevention, and psychosocial function. A discussion regarding algorithms as clinical tools appears in Chapter 2 of this handbook.

Individuals' responses to treatment and the threat of recurrence are contingent on the type and stage of a primary malignancy. A risk stratification approach can help to address each survivor's unique, complex needs. McCabe and colleagues described risk-based care as "a personalized systematic plan of periodic screening, surveillance, and prevention relevant to the cancer experience" (14).

MD Anderson has developed an interdisciplinary team approach that is the foundation of algorithms for cancer survivors. This model of care addresses each patient's treatment response and recurrence threats that are contingent upon the type and stage of the primary malignancy. Age, sex, and overall health status primarily influence treatment type and may affect responses to treatment received.

Care for cancer survivors should be tiered based upon risk factors and degree of care required. Figure 1.3 provides an example of each tier.

- Tier 1: Patients in this group are at low risk for complications or recurrence. The aims of care are symptom management, smoking-cessation counseling, energy balance, and healthy living
- Tier 2: These patients are at risk for late effects of treatment; they have received combined-modality therapies including chemotherapy, radiation, and surgery. This subgroup is at higher risk for secondary cancers, and primary care providers and oncologists should comanage follow-up care
- Tier 3: Patients in this category are at high risk if they experience a cancer reoccurrence or late effects from their treatment. Patients who undergo stem-cell transplantation, for example, fall into this tier. These patients should be followed closely by an oncologist and primary care provider to manage comorbid conditions and health issues

As providers in a major comprehensive cancer center with 12 disease-specific clinics, clinicians at MD Anderson have established survivorship care from a unique

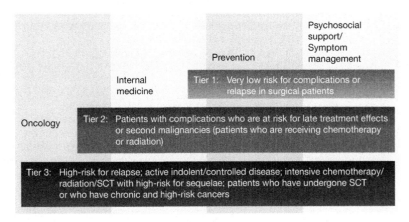

FIGURE 1.3 Stratified tiers of medical risk.
SCT, stem cell transplantation.

perspective. Clinical, educational, and research aspects are combined to provide high-quality survivorship care. Care for long-term survivors must be tailored to each patient. Models of care delivery can vary in their operational structure but must be clinically designed to optimally address complication risks and include the key IOM domains for the delivery of survivorship care: surveillance, prevention, monitoring for late effects, and psychosocial health. Healthcare providers must deliver care based on individual survivor needs.

The number of cancer survivors continue to increase. The aim of survivorship care is to address the impact of cancer care and its therapies in an effort to improve survivors' health and quality of life. Therefore, care for long-term survivors must be tailored to each patient. Models of care delivery are most optimal when they address complication risk while including the key domains of surveillance, prevention, monitoring of late effects, and psychosocial health.

REFERENCES

1. Institute of Medicine. *From Cancer Patient to Cancer Survivor—Lost in Transition: An American Society of Clinical Oncology and Institute of Medicine symposium.* Washington, DC: National Academies Press; 2006.
2. Marzorati C, Riva S, Pravettoni G. Who is a cancer survivor? A systematic review of published definitions. *J Cancer Educ.* 2017;32(2):228–237. doi:10.1007/s13187-016-0997-2
3. National Cancer Institute. Survivorship. NCI dictionary of cancer terms. Available at: https://www.cancer.gov/publications/dictionaries/cancer-terms?cdrid=445089
4. de Moor JS, Mariotto AB, Parry C, et al. Cancer survivors in the United States: prevalence across the survivorship trajectory and implications for care. *Cancer Epidemiol Biomarkers Prev.* 2013;22(4):561–570. doi:10.1158/1055-9965.EPI-12-1356
5. Miller KD, Siegel RL, Lin CC, et al. Cancer treatment and survivorship statistics, 2016. *CA Cancer J Clin.* 2016;66(4):271–289. doi:10.3322/caac.21349
6. Siegel RL, Miller KD, Jemal A. Cancer statistics, 2017. *CA Cancer J Clin.* 2017;67(1):7–30. doi:10.3322/caac.21395
7. Mullan F. Seasons of survival: reflections of a physician with cancer. *N Engl J Med.* 1985;313(4):270–273. doi:10.1056/NEJM198507253130421
8. Mayer DK, Nasso SF, Earp JA. Defining cancer survivors, their needs, and perspectives on survivorship health care in the USA. *Lancet Oncol.* 2017;18(1):e11–e18. doi:10.1016/S1470-2045(16)30573-3
9. Institute of Medicine. *Delivering High-Quality Cancer Care: Charting a New Course for a System in Crisis.* Washington, DC: National Academies Press; 2013.
10. Commission on Cancer. Chapter 3: Continuum of care services. In: *Cancer Program Standards: Ensuring Patient-Centered Care.* 2016:54–58. Available at: https://www.facs.org/~/media/files/quality%20programs/cancer/coc/2016%20coc%20standards%20manual_interactive%20pdf.ashx
11. Ryerson AB, Wasilewski-Masker K, Border WL, et al. Pediatric quality of life in long-term survivors of childhood cancer treated with anthracyclines. *Pediatr Blood Cancer.* 2016;63(12):2205–2211. doi:10.1002/pbc.26149

12. Shaikh F, Dupuis LL, Alexander S, et al. Cardioprotection and second malignant neoplasms associated with dexrazoxane in children receiving anthracycline chemotherapy: a systematic review and meta-analysis. *J Natl Cancer Inst*. 2016;108(4). doi:10.1093/jnci/djv357

13. van Dalen EC, Raphaël MF, Caron HN, et al. Treatment including anthracyclines versus treatment not including anthracyclines for childhood cancer. *Cochrane Database Syst Rev*. 2014(9):CD006647. doi:10.1002/14651858.CD006647.pub4

14. McCabe MS, Partridge AH, Grunfeld E, et al. Risk-based health care, the cancer survivor, the oncologist, and the primary care physician. *Semin Oncol*. 2013;40(6):804–812. doi:10.1053/j.seminoncol.2013.09.004

2 Tools and Resources to Improve Cancer Survivorship Clinical Practice and Care

Guadalupe R. Palos
Katherine R. Gilmore

In its 2005 report, *From Cancer Patient to Cancer Survivor: Lost in Transition*, the Institute of Medicine (IOM) stated that evidence-based practice knowledge is necessary to inform clinicians and patients about the best care for long-term cancer survivors (1). This report established the philosophy of best practice, outlined the basic components of survivorship care, and described the need for basic clinical tools to enhance survivorship care. Since its release, substantial progress has been made in the care of survivors, including those who have completed active treatment and are receiving long-term care (2). These advances include the emergence of new models of survivorship care (3), development of and criteria for quality clinical guidelines (4,5), and release of mandates to provide standardized care to all survivors (6). These trends underscore the importance of providing specialized care to long-term cancer survivors.

IOM CORE DOMAINS

The core elements of survivorship care were established in the IOM report; these elements include surveillance for recurrence and new primary cancers, risk reduction and health promotion, management of late and long-term effects, and coordination of care between oncologists and primary care providers (PCPs) (1). The report also emphasized the importance of appropriate resources to promote communication, coordination, and collaboration among oncologists, patients, and PCPs. Although survivorship clinical tools and educational resources are available, they often are underused or overlooked (7,8). This chapter discusses resources available for clinicians who work with survivors and includes clinical practice algorithms, survivorship care plans (SCPs), and educational resources for medical professionals and survivors and their families. A case study will illustrate the application of these tools in a multidisciplinary survivorship clinic at a large comprehensive cancer center.

CLINICAL ALGORITHMS: A HELPFUL TOOL FOR ONCOLOGISTS AND PCPs

Oncologists and other providers may not be familiar with survivorship care because it is an evolving specialty (2,9). Since the release of IOM's report, there has been an increase in clinical decision-making tools, which encourages clinicians to change their practice and implement evidence-based survivorship care. This section discusses the core elements of survivorship care and describes algorithms, which are efficient and practical tools that can be used in any type of clinical practice or setting.

Two recommendations in IOM's report called for the use of clinical tools to promote quality survivorship care (10). One recommendation advised cancer survivors to receive a treatment summary and SCP after completing active treatment. These documents can enhance coordination of care and communication among providers regarding a survivor's physical and mental health-related needs. Another IOM recommendation advocated for use of clinical pathways or algorithms to guide clinician decision making in the delivery of survivorship care (1).

Clinical practice pathways, guidelines, or algorithms are consensus or evidence-based decision tools that help to standardize clinical practice and enhance quality and coordination of care (9). Several major oncology professional organizations have developed clinical guidelines for cancer survivors (11,12). The guidelines differ according to disease site (breast, colorectal, and other selected cancers), topic (late effects such as fatigue), and structure (four IOM domains), and all are available online (Table 2.1 lists URLs). Although the tools may differ by cancer site and content, they provide a systematic method for the surveillance, treatment, and delivery of coordinated care to long-term survivors. These tools can minimize variation in care and provide quick access to the most current science in survivorship care. In this chapter, the word *algorithm* is used in a global sense to describe clinical tools that can be employed in the care of long-term cancer survivors.

TABLE 2.1 Cancer Survivorship Guideline Websites

Organization	Topics	URL
American Cancer Society	Breast cancer, colorectal cancer, prostate cancer, head and neck cancers	www.cancer.org/health-care-professionals/american-cancer-society-survivorship-guidelines.html
National Cancer Comprehensive Network		
American Society of Clinical Oncologists	Late and long-term effects including fatigue, anxiety, depressive symptoms, and peripheral neuropathy Cancer sites include prostate and breast Surveillance includes breast follow-up, colorectal cancer, gynecologic oncology	www.asco.org/practice-guide-lines/cancer-care-initiatives/prevention-survivorship/survivorship-compendium-0

(continued)

TABLE 2.1 Cancer Survivorship Guideline Websites (*continued*)

Organization	Topics	URL
Children's Oncology Group	Long-term follow-up for survivors of childhood, adolescent, and young adult cancers	www.survivorshipguidelines.org
National Comprehensive Cancer Network	Late effects/long-term effects, psychosocial and physical problems, preventive health, smoking cessation, distress management, and cancer-related fatigue	www.nccn.org/store/login/login.aspx?ReturnURL=https://www.nccn.org/professionals/physician_gls/pdf/survivorship.pdf (Must register for an account, and guideline access is free)

Algorithms, guidelines, and pathways encourage value-based oncology care, decrease inappropriate care, promote personalized care, and improve overall quality of care for patients (9). Cancer survivors also benefit because use of these tools can facilitate better communication between patients and providers, increase patient engagement, and enhance shared decision making (13).

TREATMENT SUMMARIES AND SCPs: ESSENTIAL ELEMENTS

The cornerstones of survivorship care are the treatment summary and SCP. These documents should include details about treatment received; timing and content of recommended follow-up; preventive practices; and information related to employment, insurance, and psychosocial resources. These documents are intended to enhance communication, collaboration, and coordination of care among oncologists, PCPs, and survivors. It is important to note that although clinicians use this tool in their practice, the content and format should be designed so that patients can also use the document to track their follow-up care.

The Commission on Cancer (COC) released 2012 standards that require all cancer treatment facilities to provide a treatment summary and follow-up care plan to patients who complete their treatment with curative intent (6). The COC mandate also requires that these documents be given to survivors within 12 months after diagnosis and no longer than 6 months after completion of adjuvant therapy (or 18 months from diagnosis if the patient receives hormonal therapy) (6).

Since the early 2000s, several professional organizations, including the National Comprehensive Cancer Network, American Cancer Society, American Society of Clinical Oncologists (ASCO), CancerNet, and others, have released SCP templates (14). The purpose of an SCP is to personalize and coordinate care by sharing the document with the survivors' other healthcare providers. These tools vary in length, content, and delivery method, and most are web-based and available to all professionals and to the public (Table 2.2).

In 2011, leading survivorship experts convened a national conference to reach a consensus on the core elements needed for any SCP. These elements are grouped into three tiers; importance is ranked as acknowledged through the consensus process (Figure 2.1) (15).

TABLE 2.2 Survivorship Care Plan Templates Available Online

Organization	URL
American Cancer Society	www.cancer.org/treatment/survivorship-during-and-after-treatment/survivorship-care-plans.html
American Society of Clinical Oncologists	www.cancer.net/survivorship/follow-care-after-cancer-treatment/asco-cancer-treatment-and-survivorship-care-plans
Journey Forward	www.journeyforward.org/professionals/survivorship-care-plan-builder
LIVESTRONG/OncoLife	oncolife.oncolink.org/form/oncolife_v11

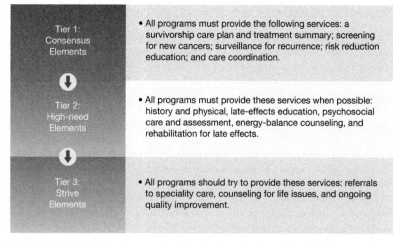

FIGURE 2.1 Essential elements of survivorship cancer care.
Source: Adapted from Rechis R, Beckjord B, Avery et al. *The Essential Elements of Survivorship Care: A LIVESTRONG Brief.* LIVESTRONG Foundation; December 2011. Available at: https://d1un1nybq8gi3x.cloudfront.net/sites/default/files/what-we-do/reports/EssentialElementsBrief.pdf.

A CASE STUDY AT MD ANDERSON'S SURVIVORSHIP CLINIC

At MD Anderson, survivors may choose the ways in which they receive their follow-up care after completing treatment. Survivors may choose to return to their community for follow-up care (option 1) with a PCP who communicates with the treating oncologist when and if needed. Other survivors may choose to stay at the treatment institution and transition to a survivorship clinic that is appropriate for their disease site (option 2). On occasion, a survivor cannot be transitioned because a survivorship clinic is not available for their particular type of cancer. These survivors are followed in their primary oncology clinic by their treating physician (option 3).

Transitioning to Survivorship Care

Oncologists, internists, family practice physicians, and midlevel clinicians (advanced nurse practitioners and physician assistants) are the primary providers in MD Anderson's survivorship clinics. Survivors typically are seen in the survivorship clinic on an annual basis by the same provider.

A clinic visit includes a history and physical examination; a detailed assessment of changes in the survivor's physical and psychosocial functioning, including potential symptoms of recurrent or new primary cancers or comorbid conditions; cancer screening recommendations tailored to the individual survivor; assessment for late treatment effects; a nutrition assessment and counseling; consultation or referrals for support services; and a personalized follow-up care plan. Once a survivor is transitioned to a survivorship clinic, a clinician can use its institutional tools (i.e., algorithms, treatment summaries, and care plans) to provide follow-up care.

The Road Map to Long-Term Survivor Care

A clinical algorithm is the road map that guides clinicians and survivors through a survivorship clinic visit. Survivorship algorithms are designed to provide a visual and written guide to support providers' delivery of quality care. The structure and clinical process outlined in Figure 2.2 serve as the standard foundation for all algorithms regardless of disease site. Each algorithm has these components: eligibility criteria; clinical strategies, interventions, procedures, and recommendations (related to surveillance, risk reduction and early detection, monitoring for late effects, and psychosocial functioning); and potential visit outcomes. Algorithms summarize the necessary procedures, tests, counseling, and education for each of four IOM domains and are tailored to specific cancer sites.

Each algorithm begins with a list of eligibility criteria specific to a disease site (Figure 2.2). By using these criteria, a clinician can confirm whether the survivorship clinic is appropriate for a survivor. The next step in the algorithm focuses on surveillance of a survivor's risk for a new primary cancer or recurrence of the original cancer. The assessment allows the provider to focus on risk-reduction/early detection recommendations specific to a survivors' health needs. The provider may also include patient counseling and education on screening procedures (breast and colorectal cancer),

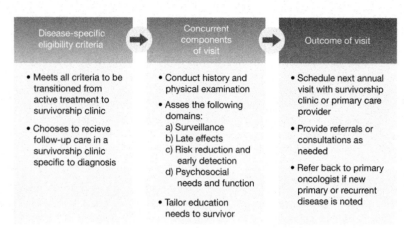

FIGURE 2.2 Conceptual framework used for each survivorship care algorithm. Specific content and decision points were presented in narrative and visual formats (decision-tree flow graphic). Algorithms are available at www.mdanderson.org/for-physicians/clinical-tools-resources/clinical-practice-algorithms/survivorship-algorithms.html.

energy-balance activities (weight management, exercise), smoking cessation guidelines, and sun exposure. The next algorithm step concentrates on monitoring for late effects. Based on the type of cancer, its stage, and treatment type the survivor received, a provider can tailor assessment, management, counseling, and education for late effects. The last part of the algorithm focuses on assessment of a survivor's psychosocial functioning. The provider also can assess a survivor's distress level, social support networks, and need for other types of interventions. At times, a survivor may need a referral for a more in-depth consultation with a social worker, psychiatrist, or community-based mental health provider.

Delivery of Personalized Survivorship Care

At the end of the visit, each survivor receives a personalized two-page treatment summary and care plan to share with their primary provider (Figure 2.3). The form consists of a treatment summary and care plan. The same template is used for each clinic; however, recommendations are tailored to each site-specific cancer.

To accommodate different learning preferences, the algorithms are provided in narrative and graphical formats. Figure 2.4 is an example of a template used in a comprehensive cancer center for each survivorship algorithm. To date, MD Anderson has developed 47 clinical practice algorithms for 11 adult survivorship clinics. Once eligibility is confirmed, an algorithm outlines steps needed to address the full spectrum

Patient Demographics — Page 1

Patient name: _____ DOB: _____

Health care providers (surgeon, radiation oncologist, medical oncologist, additional cancer providers):

Cancer diagnosis (date, stage, histology, tumor markers):

Cancer treatment history:

Surgery
☐ Yes   ☐ No

Date	Procedure
Primary surgery:	
Reconstruction:	
Other:	

Chemotherapy
☐ Yes   ☐ No

Date completed	Treatment indicated	Drug name(s)	Cycles

Radiation therapy
☐ Yes   ☐ No

Date completed	Primary or postoperative	Type/site tool	Dose	Number of fractions

Cancer surveillance and screening — Page 2

Provide recommendations for when and whom (oncologist or primary care) will perform the following:

Surveillance	When	Where
• Imaging surveillance for recurrence of primary cancer (e.g., CT, MRI, mammography, colonoscopy, ultrasound)		
• Laboratory test for tumor markers (e.g., PSA, CA125)		

Late effects/side effects management

Counsel patient on potential late or long-term side effects

Provide referrals to screen for or manage ongoing late effects such as:

Late effect	Recommendation
• Bone health, cardiac dysfunction, lymphedema, sexual health/fertility, fatigue, neuropathy, cognitive dysfunction	

Risk reduction and cancer prevention

Provide recommendations for when and whom (oncologist or primary care) will perform the following:

Preventive screening	When	Where
• Gynecologic screening, colorectal screening, breast screening, prostate screening, skin screening, lung cancer screening, and genetic screening.		

Counsel on behavioral risk reduction strategies. Provide recommendations pertinent to patient:

Risk reduction	Recommendation
• Smoking cessation, weight loss, exercise/physical activity, diet, vaccinations	

Psychosocial functioning

Asses for and provide referrals for psychosocial issues related to cancer and its treatment, including:

	Recommendation
• Distress, financial issues, body image concerns, social support concerns	

FIGURE 2.3 Survivorship care plan template used at a comprehensive cancer center.

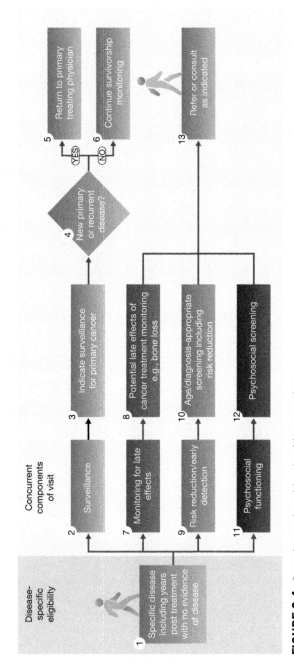

FIGURE 2.4 Generic survivorship algorithm template.

of care. The tools are designed to be easily retrieved, stored, and displayed through institutional clinical information systems and printed sources. Clinicians can access algorithms in print or electronic formats that include clinic binders, web-based clinical portals, and the Intranet/Internet. Survivors can also access the algorithms through a link provided on the survivorship program website.

To enhance clinician engagement (oncologists, internists, family practice physicians, advanced nurse practitioners, and physician assistants), educational in-service trainings are provided on how to use an algorithm as a road map for a survivorship clinic visit. Clinicians also have support from a project consultant who specializes in the setup of survivorship clinics, implementation of algorithms, and clinic codes for reimbursement of survivorship care. The project consultant provides ongoing support and education to clinicians on the best practice for implementation of the algorithms and coordination of care.

Shift From Surveillance to Survivorship and Training

Education must shift from surveillance to survivorship as cancer survivors live longer. This phase of the cancer continuum represents the new "teachable moment" for clinician–survivor discussions about the value of SCPs and follow-up care (16).

Adequate training and education for oncologists, PCPs, and oncology nurses must be available to meet the needs of long-term cancer survivors (2,17,18). Fortunately, educational opportunities for oncologists and PCPs focused on survivorship care of long-term survivors are increasing. ASCO and other independent organizations offer specific curriculums, graduate medical education, and scientific conferences and professional development courses to address the broad needs of long-term survivors. The development and dissemination of evidence-based guidelines also supports the educational needs of medical professionals such as those involved in primary medicine residency programs (19). Integration of survivorship care into academic curricula in medicine, nursing, physical therapy, psychology, nutrition, and other disciplines can help to prepare the new cadre of medical professionals to care for long-term cancer survivors.

Healthcare professionals will benefit from building collaborative networks with nononcology specialties because of the broad nature the survivors' medical and psychological, preventive, and supportive care needs (i.e., regarding care-related costs and employment concerns) (20,21). Survivors' follow-up visits will involve a history and physical (22); assessment of late and long-term effects; surveillance of symptoms to detect new or recurrent cancers; a discussion of risk-reduction activities such as screenings for breast, colorectal, prostate, and gynecological cancers; and primary prevention health promotion education on topics such as smoking cessation, nutritional needs, or physical activities (23). Referrals to local resources will help survivors access these types of services.

Educational Resources for Survivors, Caregivers, and Their Families

Opportunities for "teachable moments" occur when survivors, caregivers, and their family members receive information and education that meets their immediate needs and concerns. Knowledge regarding risky health behaviors, later and long-term effects for which monitoring is required, and recommended screening tests can foster survivors' self-management of their care (24). Numerous websites offer survivorship care educational resources (Table 2.3). Other organizations provide online services related to finances, psychosocial support, caregiver needs, and other areas that can influence the lives of long-term cancer survivors. These educational resources are available in many different languages.

Quality survivorship care can be delivered when medical professionals, survivors, and their families combine and use their knowledge to address the complex issues affecting care of long-term cancer survivors.

TABLE 2.3 Survivorship Care Web-Based Educational Resources

Organization	URL
American Society of Clinical Oncologists Survivorship care educational opportunities provide links to courses, meetings, position statements, and other valuable resources for healthcare professionals interested in survivorship care.	www.asco.org/practice-guide-lines/cancer-care-initiatives/prevention-survivorship/survivorship/survivorship-9
Centers for Disease Control and Prevention The steps and programs underway to examine the health concerns of survivors using a public health approach are outlined. Segments provide basic information on SCPs for healthcare professionals, researchers, caregivers, and patients. Web Plus Survivorship Module (helps practitioners improve cancer survivorship care planning).	www.cdc.gov/cancer/survivorship www.cdc.gov/cancer/npcr/tools/registryplus/wp_survmodule.htm
George Washington University Cancer Institute and the American Cancer Society National Cancer Survivorship Resource Center Toolkit: Implementing Clinical Practice Guidelines for Cancer Survivorship Care.	smhs.gwu.edu/gwci/sites/gwci/files/NCSRC%20Toolkit%20FINAL.pdf?src=GWCI
National Cancer Institute Office of Cancer Survivorship, Division of Cancer Control and Population Sciences Survivorship-related definitions, resources, statistics, and news are available at this website.	cancercontrol.cancer.gov/ocs
The University of Texas MD Anderson Cancer Center The Cancer Survivorship Series offers several courses focusing on basics of survivorship care to advanced courses on care of site-specific cancers.	www.mdanderson.org/education-training/professional-education/professional-oncology-education/survivorship.html

SCPs, survivorship care plans.

REFERENCES

1. Institute of Medicine. *From Cancer Patient to Cancer Survivors: Lost in Transition.* Washington, DC: National Academies Press; 2006.
2. McCabe MS, Bhatia S, Oeffinger KC, et al. American Society of Clinical Oncology statement: achieving high-quality cancer survivorship care. *J Clin Oncol.* 2013;31(5):631–640.
3. McCabe MS, Jacobs LA. Clinical update: survivorship care—models and programs. *Semin Oncol Nurs.* 2012;28(3):e1–e8.
4. Abrahams E, Balch A, Goldsmith P, et al. Clinical pathways: recommendations for putting patients at the center of value-based care. *Clin Cancer Res.* 2017;23(16):1–5.
5. Zon RT, Edge SB, Page RD, et al. American Society of Clinical Oncology criteria for high-quality clinical pathways in oncology. *J Oncol Pract.* 2017;13(3):207–210.
6. American College of Surgeons and Commission on Cancer. Cancer Program Standards 2012: Ensuring Patient-Centered Care. Available at: https://www.facs.org/~/media/files/quality%20programs/cancer/coc/programstandards2012updates.ashx. Published in 2011.
7. Birken SA, Mayer DK, Weiner BJ. Survivorship care plans: prevalence and barriers to use. *J Cancer Educ.* 2013;28(2):290–296.
8. Jacobs LA, Shulman LN. Follow-up care of cancer survivors: challenges and solutions. *Lancet Oncol.* 2017;18(1):e19–e29.
9. Nekhlyudov L, O'malley DM, Hudson SV. Integrating primary care providers in the care of cancer survivors: gaps in evidence and future opportunities. *Lancet Oncol.* 2017;18(1):e30–e38.
10. Grant M, Economou D, Ferrell B, et al. Educating health care professionals to provide institutional changes in cancer survivorship care. *J Cancer Educ.* 2012;27(2):226–232.
11. Cohen EE, LaMonte SJ, Erb NL, et al. American Cancer Society head and neck cancer survivorship care guideline. *CA Cancer J Clin.* 2016;66(3):203–239.
12. Ligibel JA, Denlinger CS. New NCCN guidelines(R) for survivorship care. *J Natl Compr Canc Netw.* 2013;11(suppl 5):640–644.
13. Chawla A, Westrich K, Matter S, Kaltenboeck A, Dubois R. Care pathways in US healthcare settings: current successes and limitations, and future challenges. *Am J Manag Care.* 2016;22(1):53–62.
14. Hahn EE, Ganz PA. Survivorship programs and care plans in practice: variations on a theme. *J Oncol Pract.* 2011;7(2):70–75.
15. Rechis R, Beckjord B, Avery SR, et al. *The Essential Elements of Survivorship Care: A LIVESTRONG Brief.* LIVESTRONG Foundation; December 2011. Available at: https://d1un1nybq8gi3x.cloudfront.net/sites/default/files/what-we-do/reports/EssentialElementsBrief.pdf
16. Flocke SA, Clark E, Antognoli E, et al. Teachable moments for health behavior change and intermediate patient outcomes. *Patient Educ Couns.* 2014;96(1):43–49.
17. Shapiro CL, Jacobsen PB, Henderson T, et al. ReCAP: ASCO core curriculum for cancer survivorship education. *J Oncol Pract.* 2016;12(2):145, e108–e117.
18. Palos GR, Lewis-Patterson P, Gilmore K, et al. Changing nursing practice in survivorship care with clinical decision tools. *Clin J Oncol Nurs.* 2015;19(4):482–484, 488.
19. Susanibar S, Thrush CR, Khatri N, et al. Cancer survivorship training: a pilot study examining the educational gap in primary care medicine residency programs. *J Cancer Surviv.* 2014;8(4):565–570.

20. Pandey P, Barber F. Improving the education and training of primary care nurse practitioners to meet the healthcare needs of long-term cancer survivors. *Clin J Oncol Nurs.* 2016;20(3):334–335.

21. Lewis-Patterson P, Palos GR, Dains J, et al. Cancer prevention in the survivorship setting. *Semin Oncol Nurs.* 2016;32(3):291–305.

22. Fuentes AC, Lambird JE, George TJ Jr, et al. Cancer survivor's history and physical. *South Med J.* 2017;110(1):37–44.

23. Sisler J, Chaput G, Sussman J, et al. Follow-up after treatment for breast cancer: practical guide to survivorship care for family physicians. *Can Fam Physician.* 2016;62(10):805–811.

24. Lajous M, Mozaffarian D, Mozaffarian R, et al. Lifestyle prescriptions for cancer survivors and their communities. *J Intern Med.* 2011;269(1):88–93.

3

Late and Long-Term Effects in Cancer Survivors

Jeong Hoon Oh

Late effects are prolonged health effects that are absent or subclinical during the treatment period and that manifest after the end of the treatment responsible for the health effect. *Long-term effects* are prolonged health effects that manifest during the treatment responsible for the health effect and continue after discontinuation of treatment.

This chapter addresses some of the most serious physical late and long-term effects. Psychosocial late effects and secondary cancers will be addressed in Chapters 4 and 5 and in site-specific chapters.

BACKGROUND

A steady increase in cancer survivorship during recent decades has surpassed increases in the incidence of many chronic conditions including peptic ulcer disease, coronary artery disease (CAD), stroke, chronic obstructive pulmonary disease, and chronic kidney disease. Factors that contribute to cancer treatment success include new chemotherapy formulations and schedules that allow higher total dosages, aggressive chemotherapy with stem cell rescue, targeted immunotherapy, novel surgical techniques, and use of multimodality treatment.

Improved cancer treatment outcomes, however, are associated with an increase in the number of patients and survivors who are affected by the late effects of cancer treatment. Studies suggest that as many as 20% of primary care physician (PCP) patient rosters include cancer survivors. However, PCPs say they do not feel comfortable screening for or managing late cancer effects (1).

Late Effects: Functional Status and Prevalence

Survivors with late effects experience impaired mental and physical health and high use of health services and report more unmet health needs than survivors without late effects. By age 50, childhood cancer survivors have a 53.6% cumulative incidence of fatal, life-threatening, severe, or disabling health conditions when compared with their sibling control group (19.8%) (2). In another study comparing childhood cancer survivors with siblings without cancer, cancer survivors were at increased risk for major joint replacement, congestive heart failure, and CAD (3). Results of a 2010 Livestrong Foundation voluntary web-based survey of cancer survivors suggest that some late effects of cancer and treatment may lead to substantial functional impairment. For example, only 16% of survivors with fatigue, 18% with pain, 47% with lymphedema, and 54% with neuropathy reported that late effects did not lead to functional impairment (4).

Prevalence of individual late effects can vary substantially based upon cancer type and treatment received. Published rates in systematic reviews range from 4% (cardiac events after surgery and chemotherapy) to 65% (erectile dysfunction after prostatectomy) (5). As a general principle, combination treatment with radiation and chemotherapy leads to higher incidence of late effects in radiated areas (this is particularly applicable regarding cardiovascular effects).

Cardiovascular Late Effects

Cardiac dysfunction/cardiomyopathy traditionally is associated with use of anthracyclines, antimetabolites, and alkylating agents such as cyclophosphamide. However, other chemotherapeutic agents such as taxanes (paclitaxel and docetaxel) and, more recently, targeted therapies such as vascular endothelial growth factor (VEGF) inhibitors (i.e., bevacizumab), multikinase inhibitors (i.e., sorafenib and sunitinib), and human epidermal growth factor receptor 2 (HER2) inhibitors (i.e., trastuzumab and pertuzumab) can cause left ventricular dysfunction. If the heart is in the radiation field, high-dose radiotherapy (RT; ≥30 Gy) alone or even low-dose RT (<30 Gy) in combination with use of an anthracycline has also been associated with increased risk for cardiac dysfunction.

The mechanism of anthracycline cardiotoxicity is believed to involve a topoisomerase-2b–dependent reactive oxygen species leading to oxidative damage to cardiac myocytes; direct injury to mitochondrial DNA; dysregulation of cardiac transcription; and disruption of the sarcomeric protein, titin. Heart failure risk is highest for patients who are younger than age 5 or older than age 65 at exposure and for those who have preexisting conditions and a history that includes chest radiation. The heart failure rate has decreased dramatically with the use of lower cumulative doses (reduced to 3%–5% with 400 mg/m^2 from as high as 48% with 700 mg/m^2 of doxorubicin) and also with liposomal preparations. Anthracycline cardiomyopathy may be apparent within weeks, but it also may be subclinical for decades.

Cardiomyopathy incidence resulting from cyclophosphamide (an alkylating agent) use is between 7% and 33%. Cardiomyopathy is not related to cumulative dosing but occurs more frequently with higher individual doses frequently used in autologous stem cell rescue protocols (6,7). The mechanism of action remains unclear.

HER2 inhibitors are present in cardiac myocytes and play a cardioprotective role. Animal models with cardiac restricted knockout of erbB-2 (the animal equivalent to human HER2) present with a cardiomyopathic phenotype. Cardiomyopathy resulting from trastuzumab use can occur in 1% to 4% of patients and is reversible for many patients (8). Some studies of patients with metastatic breast cancer suggest that those who develop cardiomyopathy can be rechallenged safely. Trastuzumab can potentiate cardiotoxic effects of anthracyclines (not observed with pertuzumab), but fatal cardiac events are rare.

Bevacizumab and multikinase inhibitor use, on the other hand, may lead to reversible myocyte dysfunction or cardiomyopathy through new onset of worsening hypertension, but use does not cause direct myocardial injury. Bevacizumab can cause symptomatic systolic heart failure in 2% of patients, but the rate of cardiomyopathy with multikinase inhibitor use varies with sunitinib, leading to heart failure for 8% of patients whereas agents such as afatinib are not associated with cardiotoxicity (9,10). A recently published American Society of Clinical Oncology (ASCO) clinical practice guideline, *Prevention and Monitoring of Cardiac Dysfunction in Survivors of Adult Cancers,* identified these patient groups to be at high risk for cardiac dysfunction:

1. Treatment that includes any of the following:
   - High-dose anthracycline (e.g., doxorubicin ≥ 250 mg/m^2, epirubicin ≥ 600 mg/m^2)
   - High-dose RT (≥ 30 Gy) when the heart is in the treatment field
   - Lower dose anthracycline (e.g., doxorubicin <250 mg/m^2, epirubicin <600 mg/m^2) in combination with lower-dose RT (<30 Gy) when the heart is in the treatment field.
2. Treatment with lower dose anthracycline (e.g., doxorubicin <250 mg/m^2, epirubicin <600 mg/m^2), or trastuzumab alone and the presence of any of the following risk factors:
   - Two or more cardiovascular risk factors, including smoking, hypertension, diabetes, dyslipidemia, and obesity, during or after completion of therapy
   - Older age (≥ 60 years) at cancer treatment
   - Compromised cardiac function (e.g., borderline low left ventricular ejection fraction [50%–55%], history of myocardial infarction, moderate valvular heart disease) at any time before or during treatment.
3. Treatment with lower dose anthracycline (e.g., doxorubicin <250 mg/m^2, epirubicin <600 mg/m^2) followed by trastuzumab (sequential therapy) (11).

Patients who are considered at high risk for cardiac dysfunction should be screened for modifiable cardiovascular risk factors prior to treatment initiation. Baseline and posttreatment echocardiograms (or cardiac MRI) may be needed. For cancer survivors, the most important steps in screening for cardiac dysfunction are to obtain a detailed history and perform a physical examination. For survivors with symptoms of cardiac dysfunction, further testing with imaging studies (echocardiogram, cardiac MRI, or multigated acquisition scan) should be considered.

Once a cardiac dysfunction diagnosis is established, treatment that follows evidence-based guidelines for treatment of systolic heart failure of other etiologies should be initiated. Consider referral to a provider with onco-cardiology expertise.

Radiation can lead to heart valve thickening, fibrosis, and calcification. Both stenosis and regurgitation can coexist; however, clinically significant disease usually takes 10 to 20 years to develop. Radiation to the spine most frequently is associated with injury to the tricuspid valve, and mediastinal radiation most often is associated with aortic valve damage. Patients who receive radiation to the chest or thoracic spine should be followed for signs of valvular disease for the remainder of their lives. An echocardiogram is the diagnostic test of choice. Treatment for valvular disorders resulting from cancer treatment is similar to treatment for valvular disease originating from other etiologies. However, surgical treatment can be challenging for these patients.

Pericarditis is a common effect of radiation; however, with the introduction of new techniques that reduce cardiac exposure and influence dosing schedules, pericardial disease incidence may be decreasing. There is a paucity of long-term studies, however. Pericardial disease is more prevalent among survivors with preexisting cardiac pathologies who received adjuvant chemotherapy. Symptoms are similar to pericarditis of other etiologies. Although pericardial disease may not cause symptoms, no evidence supports use of imaging studies before symptoms develop. Medical treatment involves the use of nonsteroidal anti-inflammatory drugs, colchicine, or steroids. A 2015 study suggested that percutaneous pericardiocentesis with extended catheter drainage may be the preferred treatment for patients with substantial pericardial effusion (12).

Coronary Artery Disease

Many chemotherapeutic agents and targeted therapies can cause acute coronary syndrome through vasospasm or thrombosis. However, studies of testicular cancer survivors receiving platinum-based chemotherapy suggest an increase in CAD as a late effect (observed-to-expected ratio of 7.1 in a Dutch population) (13). Additionally, in studies of Hodgkin lymphoma survivors, anthracycline-based chemotherapy and supradiaphragmatic radiation treatment use were predictors of a significantly increased standardized mortality ratio (2.5) from myocardial infarction when compared to the general population (14). Death risk persisted over 20 years and was more pronounced in childhood cancer survivors (14). Studies suggest that endothelial damage and a high number of cardiovascular risk factors are the main mechanisms for development of atherosclerosis resulting from use of most chemotherapeutic agents. Macrovascular CAD may appear as a late effect many years after radiation treatment, and its clinical presentation is similar to CAD unrelated to radiation treatment. However, some patients receiving radiation treatment may have microvascular CAD as a long-term effect, with initial symptoms appearing only weeks after radiation.

Patients who received radiation to the chest or thoracic spine should be screened for symptoms that suggest coronary disease. There is no specific recommendation for use of electrocardiogram or imaging modalities for patients without symptoms. However, if a patient receives radiation treatment during the previous year and has typical CAD symptoms with myocardial perfusion study findings suggestive of ischemia and normal angiogram findings, a microvascular CAD diagnosis must be entertained. Treatment of therapy-related macrovascular CAD is similar to treatment for noncancer-related CAD. Patients with microvascular CAD often respond well to medical therapy.

Extracranial carotid stenosis has been described in patients receiving radiation to the neck area, and critical stenosis of the internal carotid artery may be present in as many as 13% of patients; in addition, 10-year stroke incidence is higher among patients who receive radiation only versus other treatment modalities (15). Patients with carotid bruits or a clinical presentation suggestive of transient ischemic attack or stroke should be evaluated with carotid Doppler studies or magnetic resonance angiogram. Aspirin and statins remain the treatments of choice for noncritical lesions. Carotid stent placement may be preferred over angioplasty if there is severe neck fibrosis or a history of multiple surgeries or tracheostomy attributable to surgical complications. However, the rate of restenosis is higher with stent placement.

Platinum-based compounds and taxanes may cause hypertension as a late effect, possibly through endothelial damage. Elevated blood pressure may be a long-term effect of VEGF inhibitors (i.e., bevacizumab) and tyrosine kinase inhibitors (TKI; i.e., sorafenib, sunitinib, and axitinib) and last as long as 6 months after completion of treatment. Hypertension also may be attributable to an increase in vascular resistance and microvascular rarefaction of small arterioles. Treatment choice needs to reflect a patient's potential for drug interactions if he or she still receives TKIs (avoid nondihydropyridine calcium channel blockers such as verapamil and diltiazem). In addition, caution should be exercised when selecting treatment because some antihypertensive agents such as nifedipine and carvedilol may increase VEGF levels (16).

Pulmonary Effects

A study of pulmonary late and long-term effects in survivors of childhood cancer showed that survivors at age 45 were more likely to have chronic cough, need oxygen, and have lung fibrosis and recurrent pneumonia than their siblings (17). Another study demonstrated that pulmonary events are the second-leading cause of late mortality, with a standardized mortality ratio of 8.8 (18).

Multiple chemotherapeutic agents can cause lung injury, including antimetabolites (i.e., gemcitabine and methotrexate), antitumor antibiotics (i.e., bleomycin and anthracyclines), taxanes (i.e., paclitaxel and docetaxel), platinum-based compounds (particularly oxaliplatin), and many others. Lung injury can be mediated by diverse mechanisms including release of cytokines, oxidative injury from free oxygen radicals, and cell-mediated lung injury. Acute lung injury may appear in diverse forms: bronchospasm, capillary leak syndrome, hypersensitivity pneumonitis, noncardiogenic pulmonary edema, acute respiratory distress syndrome, or interstitial pneumonitis. However, among cancer survivors, pulmonary fibrosis is the most common long-term pulmonary effect.

Radiation initially causes alveolar exudates, followed by pneumonitis and then, after several months, pulmonary fibrosis. Patients who received radiation also are at high risk for recall pneumonitis, which can occur months or years after initial radiation with certain chemotherapy agents such as doxorubicin, etoposide, gentamycin, and paclitaxel.

Cough and dyspnea are the most common symptoms of pulmonary fibrosis. By the time cancer survivors develop pulmonary fibrosis, they likely will not benefit from glucocorticosteroid therapy. Referral to a pulmonologist is recommended.

Gastrointestinal Effects

Dysphagia, the most common late effect gastrointestinal symptom, usually appears several months after radiation treatment and may be caused by altered motility attributable to nerve or muscle damage or esophageal stricture.

Dyspepsia and late gastric ulceration, which can occur within several months of treatment completion, lead to abdominal pain. Antral stenosis may occur for up to 1 year after treatment, and patients may present with nausea and vomiting. Enteritis can be a long-term or late effect. Concomitant chemotherapy increases risk for enteritis. Chemotherapy may also lead to long-term diarrhea and malabsorption.

Survivors should be screened for symptoms of late gastrointestinal effects. For patients with symptoms, endoscopy or colonoscopy may be needed. Anorectal ulceration is the most common late effect, but anal stricture and incontinence also can occur. Patients with esophageal strictures may require dietary modification and referral to a gastroenterologist for endoscopic dilation. Proton pump inhibitors may help decrease recurrence of esophageal strictures after dilation. Dyspepsia and gastric ulceration may be treated with proton pump inhibitors, but histamine 2 blockers may be a better option for survivors with chronic hypomagnesemia resulting from chemotherapy or those with renal insufficiency. Antiemetics may be needed to treat nausea or vomiting. A referral to surgery may be required for gastric outlet obstruction. Treatment of enteritis should be tailored to the presenting symptoms. Patients with diarrhea may benefit from a low-fiber diet, antidiarrheal agents, and bile sequestrants. Surgery may be necessary but can be more challenging for patients who received radiation to the abdominal area because of adhesions and associated higher complication rates. Sphincter dilation and, less frequently, colostomy may be required to address severe anorectal strictures and stenosis.

Neurological Effects

Chemotherapy-induced peripheral neuropathy (CIPN) is a common long-term effect, and a 2014 systematic review reported that CIPN was present in 30% of survivors after chemotherapy (19). CIPN is associated with decreased quality of life, reduced functional ability, increased risk for falls, and higher healthcare costs. Neuropathy is associated with use of vinca alkaloids, platinum-based compounds (i.e., cisplatin, oxaliplatin, and carboplatin), microtubule stabilizing agents (i.e., paclitaxel, docetaxel, and ixabepilone), protease inhibitors (bortezomib), and systemic immunomodulators (i.e., thalidomide and lenalidomide). The mechanisms of action are manifold for each chemotherapy. For example, platinum-based compounds accumulate in dorsal root ganglion and lead to sensory neuron death through platinum-DNA adducts. Taxanes and bortezomib produce overpolymerization of microtubules, leading to disruption of axonal transports. Vinca alkaloids bind tubulin and interfere with mitotic spindle.

Clinical presentation can vary from tingling and numbness to neuropathic pain and occur in a stocking-glove distribution. Neuropathy may be associated with a decreased ability to handle small objects, worsening handwriting, and frequent drops and falls. Upon examination, there may be a loss of deep tendon reflexes (resulting from vinca alkaloid use).

History and timing of symptom onset resulting from the potentially causative chemotherapy are the most important factors contributing to CIPN. Nerve conduction studies can confirm the presence of neuropathy but cannot differentiate CIPN from other etiologies. ASCO guidelines recommend serotonin–norepinephrine reuptake inhibitors such as duloxetine and venlafaxine for CIPN treatment (20). Even though duloxetine has been more extensively studied and is associated with fewer side effects, for breast cancer survivors receiving tamoxifen, venlafaxine may be preferable because it is associated with fewer drug interactions. Use of gabapentinoids remains controversial, but these drugs may be an option for survivors with neuropathic pain, particularly if they also have diabetic neuropathy. However, renal function should be checked and the dose adjusted accordingly. Another potential option under evaluation is alpha-lipoic acid, but thyroid function must be followed because it may cause autoimmune thyroiditis and hypothyroidism.

Orthostatic hypotension, the most common autonomic dysfunction late effect, may be related to radiation treatment or surgery in the neck area, but it also has been described in association with chemotherapy treatment. Vinca alkaloids and bortezomib are the most common causative agents, but platinum-based compounds, taxanes, and thalidomide also can cause orthostatic hypotension (21). A history of CIPN often is present. The symptoms can be intermittent, lasting for several weeks to months followed by similar periods without orthostasis. Any survivor with a history of postural dizziness and falls should be screened for orthostasis. Screening may need to be repeated because of the intermittent nature of the disease. This is a diagnosis of exclusion, and other causative possibilities must be ruled out, particularly medications. Noninvasive autonomic testing such as beat-to-beat blood pressure and heart rate changes assessed with the Valsalva maneuver can be performed to help differentiate hypovolemia from other causes. Nerve conduction studies are helpful only for concomitant neuropathy diagnosis because normal results do not rule out autonomic dysfunction caused by small fibers.

Treatment is based on symptoms and is similar to treatment of orthostatic hypotension attributable to any other cause. Survivors and caregivers should be taught how to take blood pressure readings and evaluate for orthostasis to allow for easier adjustments to the treatment regimen. The first step is behavioral modification to avoid falls. Fludrocortisone and midodrine may be used, but fludrocortisone may be preferred for survivors who have cardiovascular comorbidities because midodrine is a vasoconstrictor.

Cognitive Effects

Cognitive impairment is a common long-term effect of chemotherapy and radiation treatments. Chemotherapy-induced cognitive dysfunction has been described in 17% to 78% of survivors and is associated with lower performance in memory and information processing speed for as long as 20 years after initial treatment (22). Because cognitive effects are long-term, survivors likely will undergo baseline neurocognitive testing; this testing may also be helpful for patients who did not receive a cognitive impairment diagnosis during treatment. Many studies that have evaluated imaging modalities lack diagnostic value in clinical practice. Pharmacologic interventions have been studied with mixed results; overall, methylphenidate, donepezil, memantine, and melatonin are generally well tolerated. Neuropsychological rehabilitation may be considered with the goal of maximizing function.

Metabolic Effects

Radiation is the most common cause of hypothyroidism, and a long-term (20 years) study of Hodgkin's disease survivors revealed risk exceeding 50% for this condition among survivors who received more than 45 Gy of radiation. Several targeted therapies are associated with hypothyroidism. With TKI use (i.e., sorafenib, sunitinib, axitinib, and erlotinib), hypothyroidism is a common late effect, occurring in 85% of survivors, and the mean time to development is 50 weeks after sunitinib use (23). More recently, it has been shown that checkpoint inhibitors such as ipilimumab and pembrolizumab can cause hypothyroidism (24). One mechanism is through hypophysitis and the second is via autoimmune thyroiditis with a short period of hyperthyroidism followed by prolonged hypothyroidism. Symptoms are similar to hypothyroidism of any other etiology. Patients who receive radiation to the neck area, TKIs, and checkpoint inhibitors should be screened regularly with a thyroid-stimulating hormone and free T4 laboratory studies. There is no clinical indication to follow T3 levels. Levothyroxine replacement is the treatment of choice for hypothyroidism.

Cancer-Related Fatigue

About 30% of survivors will experience fatigue symptoms for years. Fatigue is associated with chemotherapy and targeted therapy, hormonal therapy, and radiation therapy. Comorbidities, pain, and medications may also contribute to fatigue (25). If patient history suggests risk for fatigue, assessment with the brief fatigue inventory (BFI) is recommended. If the BFI score is 1 to 3, no further assessment is needed. Patients with moderate to severe BFI scores of 4 or higher can benefit from referral to a provider with experience in cancer-related fatigue for a more focused evaluation. Cancer survivors should be evaluated for potentially reversible contributing factors. They should receive counseling about cancer-related fatigue and be encouraged to engage in moderate levels of physical activity (150 min/wk of aerobic exercise and 2–3 strength training sessions per week); reversible contributing factors should be treated. Survivors also may benefit from wakefulness agents such as modafinil, psychostimulants (i.e., methylphenidate), and vitamin D (to achieve levels ranging between 40 and 60 ng/mL).

REFERENCES

1. Oh JH, Foxhall L, Basen-Engquist K, et al. Are primary care physicians ready to care for cancer survivors? *J Gen Intern Med.* 2012;27:S122–S122.

2. Armstrong GT, Kawashima T, Leisenring W, et al. Aging and risk of severe, disabling, life-threatening, and fatal events in the childhood cancer survivor study. *J Clin Oncol.* 2014;32(12):1218–1227.

3. Oeffinger KC, Mertens AC, Sklar CA, et al. Chronic health conditions in adult survivors of childhood cancer. *N Engl J Med.* 2006;355(15):1572–1582.

4. LiveStrong. A Livestrong Report, 2010. 2010. Available at: https://d1un1nybq8gi3x. cloudfront.net/sites/default/files/what-we-do/reports/LSSurvivorSurveyReport_ final_0.pdf

5. Salz T, Baxi SS, Raghunathan N, et al. Are we ready to predict late effects? A systematic review of clinically useful prediction models. *Eur J Cancer.* 2015;51(6):758–766.

6. Braverman AC, Antin JH, Plappert MT, et al. Cyclophosphamide cardiotoxicity in bone marrow transplantation: a prospective evaluation of new dosing regimens. *J Clin Oncol.* 1991;9(7):1215–1223.

7. Gottdiener JS, Appelbaum FR, Ferrans VJ, et al. Cardiotoxicity associated with high-dose cyclophosphamide therapy. *Arch Intern Med.* 1981;141(6):758–763.

8. Vejpongsa P, Yeh ETH. Prevention of anthracycline-induced cardiotoxicity. *J Am Coll Cardiol.* 2014;64(9):938–945.

9. Choueiri TK, Mayer EL, Je Y, et al. Congestive heart failure risk in patients with breast cancer treated with bevacizumab. *J Clin Oncol.* 2011;29(6):632–638.

10. Ewer MS, Ewer SM. Cardiotoxicity of anticancer treatments: what the cardiologist needs to know. *Nat Rev Cardiol.* 2010;7(10):564–575. doi:10.1038/nrcardio.2010.121

11. Armenian SH, Lacchetti C, Lenihan D. Prevention and monitoring of cardiac dysfunction in survivors of adult cancers: American Society of Clinical Oncology Clinical Practice Guideline. *J Oncol Pract.* 2017;13(4):270–275. doi:10.1200/JOP.2016.018770

12. El Haddad D, Iliescu C, Yusuf SW, et al. Outcomes of cancer patients undergoing percutaneous pericardiocentesis for pericardial effusion. *J Am Coll Cardiol.* 2015;66(20):2269–2269.

13. Meinardi MT, Gietema JA, van der Graaf WT, et al. Cardiovascular morbidity in long-term survivors of metastatic testicular cancer. *J Clin Oncol.* 2000;18(8):1725–1732.

14. Swerdlow AJ, Higgins CD, Smith P, et al. Myocardial infarction mortality risk after treatment for Hodgkin disease: a collaborative British cohort study. *J Natl Cancer Inst.* 2007;99(3):206–214.

15. Xu J, Cao Y. Radiation-induced carotid artery stenosis: a comprehensive review of the literature. *Interv Neurol.* 2014;2(4):183–192.

16. Chen MH, Kerkelä R, Force T. Mechanisms of cardiac dysfunction associated with tyrosine kinase inhibitor cancer therapeutics. *Circulation.* 2008;118(1):84–95.

17. Dietz AC, Chen Y, Yasui Y, et al. Risk and impact of pulmonary complications in survivors of childhood cancer: a report from the childhood cancer survivor study. *Cancer.* 2016;122(23):3687–3696.

18. Armstrong GT, Liu Q, Yasui Y, et al. Late mortality among 5-year survivors of childhood cancer: a summary from the childhood cancer survivor study. *J Clin Oncol.* 2009;27(14):2328–2338.

19. Seretny M, Currie G, Sena E, et al. CN-16 incidence, prevalence and predictors of chemotherapy induced peripheral neuropathy: a systematic review and meta-analysis. *Neuro Oncol.* 2014;16(suppl 5):v49.

20. Hershman DL, Lacchetti C, Dworkin RH, et al. Prevention and management of chemotherapy-induced peripheral neuropathy in survivors of adult cancers: American Society of Clinical Oncology Clinical Practice Guideline. *J Clin Oncol.* 2014;32(18):1941–1941.

21. Park SB, Goldstein D, Krishnan AV, et al. Chemotherapy-induced peripheral neurotoxicity: a critical analysis. *CA Cancer J Clin.* 2013;63(6):419–437.

22. Schagen SB, Wefel JS. Chemotherapy-related changes in cognitive functioning. *EJC Suppl.* 2013;11(2):225–232.

23. Rini BI, Tamaskar I, Shaheen P, et al. Hypothyroidism in patients with metastatic renal cell carcinoma treated with sunitinib. *J Natl Cancer Inst.* 2007;99(1):81–83.

24. Hamnvik OP, Larsen PR, Marqusee E. Thyroid dysfunction from antineoplastic agents. *J Natl Cancer Inst.* 2011;103(21):1572–1587.

25. Bower JE, Bak K, Berger A, et al. Screening, assessment, and management of fatigue in adult survivors of cancer: An American Society of Clinical Oncology clinical practice guideline adaptation. *J Clin Oncol.* 2014;32(17):1840–U1127.

4 Psychosocial Issues

Karen Stepan
Lynn Waldmann

Cancer care today often provides state-of-the-science biomedical treatment, but fails to address the psychological and social (psychosocial) problems associated with the illness. This failure can compromise the effectiveness of health care and thereby adversely affect the health of cancer patients. Psychological and social problems created or exacerbated by cancer can cause additional suffering, weaken adherence to prescribed treatments, and threaten patients' return to health.

—Institute of Medicine [IOM] (1)

PSYCHOSOCIAL DISTRESS DEFINED

Distress has been defined as a "multifactorial, unpleasant emotional experience that extends along a continuum, ranging from common normal feelings of vulnerability, sadness and fears to problems that can be disabling such as depression, anxiety, panic, social isolation, existential and spiritual crisis" (2). Therefore, as a standard of practice, distress should be "recognized, monitored, documented and treated promptly at all stages of disease and in all settings" (2).

The National Comprehensive Cancer Center's Distress Thermometer and Problem List is a validated tool for screening for the level of distress and for the nature of the problem(s) that may accompany that distress (2). Appropriate in most settings, this tool can be used to open lines of communication between a new or seasoned survivor and his or her medical team. The tool captures the level of distress and medical and nonmedical needs as defined by the cancer survivor. If this tool is integrated into the electronic health record and a standardized process is used for its administration, practitioners' understanding of the issues faced by cancer survivors will be greatly enhanced.

THE IMPORTANCE OF ADDRESSING PSYCHOSOCIAL NEEDS

Considering the expectation that more than 40% of Americans will receive a cancer diagnosis at some point in their lifetime (1) and an estimated 30% of patients with cancer will experience substantial levels of distress at some stage of their disease trajectory (3), it is critical to address their psychosocial needs when they begin to receive care. Moreover, clinicians should assign the same level of importance and integration to psychosocial needs as to clinical care.

During the last two decades, substantial advances have been made in addressing the psychosocial consequences of cancer (4). However, many people living with cancer

TABLE 4.1 Cancer Survivor Resources

Resource	URL
American Cancer Society Cancer Survivors Network	csn.cancer.org
Cancer and Careers	www.cancerandcareers.org
CancerCare	www.cancercare.org
Cancer Legal Resource Center	cancerlegalresources.org
I'm Too Young for This! Cancer Foundation	stupidcancer.org
The Lance Armstrong Foundation	www.livestrong.org
National Cancer Institute	www.cancercontrol.cancer.gov/ocs
National Coalition for Cancer Survivorship	www.canceradvocacy.org
Patient Advocate Foundation	www.patientadvocate.org
Surviving and Moving Forward: The Samfund	www.thesamfund.org

say their psychosocial healthcare needs are not well addressed and report dissatisfaction with the amount and type of information they receive about their diagnosis, prognosis, available treatments, and ways to manage and cope with their illness (1). As a result, IOM emphasized the need for healthcare providers to address the psychological needs of patients with cancer, both through the effective detection of distress and the provision of appropriate support services before, during, and after treatment (1).

Patients with cancer often say their care providers do not understand their psychosocial needs; do not consider psychosocial support an integral part of their care; are unaware of psychosocial healthcare resources; and fail to recognize, adequately treat, and offer referrals for depression or other stress-related issues attributable to treatment of their cancer (1). Survivors may sustain permanent damage to vital organs (heart, lungs, liver, or kidneys) and experience other changes such as cognitive difficulties, fatigue, fertility issues, pain, premature aging, sexual dysfunction, and/or sleep loss (5,6). And their psychosocial health—and the health and well-being of their family members and caregivers—may decline as well. Table 4.1 features a list of resources for cancer survivors.

CANCER SURVIVORS' PSYCHOSOCIAL NEEDS

In 2015, Burg and others identified 16 themes of unmet needs among 2-, 5-, and 10-year cancer survivors (7). Unmet needs for the 1,514 survey respondents (in order of importance) were:

■ Physical needs (symptom management; sexual dysfunction; and maintaining good health with diet, exercise, and rest)

- Financial needs (affordability of services and products)
- Education and information needs (what to expect as a cancer survivor)
- Personal control needs (the ability to maintain autonomy)
- System-of-care needs (continuity of care; inadequate responses from providers)
- Resource needs (access to supplies, equipment, therapies, and medications)
- Emotional and mental health needs (fears of recurrence, new cancers, death, and dying; depression; anxiety; and negative feelings such as anger or guilt)
- Social support needs (access to support groups; use of own experiences to help others)
- Societal needs (being able to address society's response to cancer; discrimination)
- Communication needs (talking about and explaining their cancer to others)
- Provider relationship needs (trust in providers regarding decision making, follow-through, follow-up, and support)
- Cure concerns (wish/hope for a cure and effective treatments)
- Body image needs (feeling unattractive and/or ashamed)
- Survivor identity needs (identifying or not identifying as a cancer survivor)
- Employment needs (obtaining or maintaining a source of income)
- Existential/spiritual needs (being at peace in life and finding meaning in the cancer experience)

Overall, the number and type of unmet needs were not associated with the time since cancer treatment; older cancer survivors identified fewer unmet needs on average than younger survivors, and breast cancer survivors identified more unmet needs than survivors of other cancers such as prostate, colorectal, bladder, uterine, and skin. However, prostate cancer survivors identified personal control problems as a current unmet need (7).

CONSEQUENCES OF UNMET PSYCHOSOCIAL NEEDS

"Psychological comorbidity associated with cancer is linked to a range of negative health outcomes including impaired quality of life (QOL), difficulties maintaining personal and professional roles and interpersonal relationships, and impaired immune regulation and disease recovery. There is an association between distress and reduced medical compliance, prolonged hospitalization, lower levels of satisfaction with care, and higher dropout rates in clinical trials" (3). Thus, to address a cancer survivor's overall well-being, his or her needs can be categorized as practical ("daily living") needs, family needs, patient/provider communication needs, emotional needs, spiritual/religious needs, and physical needs.

Practical Needs

A cancer history can substantially influence employment opportunities and may affect a person's ability to obtain and retain health and life insurance coverage (1). Emotional anxieties about these concerns influence self-care, quality of care, and hope for the future. Resolving debt and establishing financial planning options necessitate reliable education. If a provider or medical setting cannot offer this assistance, community resources are available to help survivors make choices and take action.

Career counseling. Cancer survivors may need help enrolling in college, finding financial aid resources, exploring career and vocational opportunities, and preparing for job interviews.

Work. Return to work may come with a lack of knowledge about disability rights, privacy, confidentiality, and accommodation in the workplace. A survivor may focus on emotional concerns such as "What will people ask about my cancer?", "Can I do my old job?", and "Will my cancer history affect my employment?" These emotional concerns may interfere with the ability to effectively access information about employee protections. Information about federal employment rights, laws, job interviewing, and questions to ask or to not answer is available through community cancer resources. Cancer survivors should be encouraged to know their rights.

Insurance. Access to insurance and the ability to maintain or obtain health insurance is a major concern for survivors and their families. Cancer survivors seeking private or public insurance benefits may need assistance and information on available options.

Debt and finances. Unpaid medical bills, damaged credit, overdue taxes, and mortgage arrears are a few issues cancer survivors may encounter. Cumulative travel and lodging expenses, loss of income, copayments, prescription costs, and mounting childcare bills are additional financial hardships for survivors. These stressors can lead to feelings of inadequacy, helplessness, hopelessness, and depression. Financial experts can help cancer survivors address the present and plan for the future.

Legal. It is never too soon to prepare legal documents that will make a survivor's healthcare wishes known. Planning ahead will ensure that wishes are honored and ease the stress of decision making for loved ones.

Family Needs

Families are survivors, too. They worried and assumed multiple roles when the survivor was ill. Relationships between spouses often are affected during the cancer journey, and precancer family issues may grow more intense or heal and resolve. These issues need to be addressed for survivors and their families to enhance coping and adjustment for all.

Children. Children can "read" their family members as effectively as family members can "read" their children. Kids know when something is not normal, and their imaginary scenarios can be worse than the truth. Open communication can build trust. If children hear the cancer news from someone other than their parents or immediate family members, they may ask, "What else aren't you telling me?" Two effective MD Anderson programs address this need: Kids Inquire, We Inform (KIWI) and Children's Lives Include Moments of Bravery (CLIMB).

Talking about the journey with loved ones. Reaching out to loved ones for support during the cancer journey can allow families to grow closer and value one another more deeply. Talking about hard times helps families talk about good times.

Rebuilding roles and responsibilities. Cancer changes things. Lingering side effects from treatment may limit a survivor's ability to perform previous roles and tasks. Expressing needs, preferences, and limitations is essential to rebuild and move forward.

Patient/Provider Communication

Survivors need to feel comfortable asking questions and feel supported in their journey. Cancer survivors have unmet needs when it comes to talking about their cancer experiences with others, including their doctor, family, friends, and employers (7). The ways in which information is presented need to be clearly understood to help survivors, family members, and caregivers move forward. Diversity, cultural norms, language, spiritual belief systems, geographic regions, health literacy, and family structure/systems need to be taken into consideration when caring for survivors.

Emotional Needs

Cancer and its treatment does not only affect the body—cancer survivors may experience psychosocial, emotional, and spiritual changes. It is not easy to distinguish these changes as separate because they are so closely connected. However, these changes can affect a survivor's QOL and may linger long after treatment ends. Mental health providers are available to assist survivors with their emotions, which may include:

Anger. It is normal for a cancer survivor to be angry, especially if their anger has influenced their job, schooling, or relationships. Some survivors find it helpful to talk to a counselor or good friend or join a support group. Other survivors find it helpful to write about their anger, paint, or draw.

Anxiety and depression. Depression and anxiety are the most frequently documented disorders in adult patients with cancer—three times the prevalence rate than among the general U.S. population (3). The type of depression experienced by patients with cancer and survivors, however, is a reactive depression and is not the same as chronic depression. Some survivors come to the cancer experience with previous mental health issues that can be exacerbated by stress related to cancer. Therefore, providers should evaluate survivors' mental health at regular intervals.

Fear. Fear of recurrence is a normal and common emotional reaction upon finishing cancer treatment. No one can promise that cancer will not return.

Survivors can use coping strategies to gradually reduce fear of recurrence and help adjust to life after treatment ends.

Grief. Survivors often experience grief over multiple losses and changes resulting from their cancer, and they may miss the attention, frequency of visits, security, and support provided by the medical team. Daily QOL may diminish. As a survivor reflects on what has changed, they may experience a profound grief reaction. It is normal and healthy to mourn loss. Some survivors may need additional support to manage their grief.

Survivor guilt. In the joy of living beyond cancer, survivors may experience existential feelings and ask questions such as "Why me?" or "How come I survived and others did not?" This line of thinking sparks questions about life's uncertainty, one's place in life, personal accountability for the future, and the value one contributes. Speaking with a mental health provider may help patients process these feelings.

Spiritual/Religious Needs

Spirituality and religion often are regarded interchangeably, but for many these words have very different meanings. Religion can be defined as a specific set of beliefs and practices, usually within an organized group. Spirituality, on the other hand, is defined as a person's sense of peace, purpose, and connection to others and beliefs about the meaning of life. Many people think of themselves as spiritual, religious, or both (8).

Many cancer survivors rely on their spiritual or religious beliefs, values, and practices to help them cope with their illness. However, considering their cancer experience, they may begin to doubt their beliefs and lose faith, which can contribute to spiritual distress. Each person will have different spiritual needs depending on his or her cultural and religious traditions. Some survivors will want to talk about how cancer has influenced them spiritually but feel unsure about how to bring it up. Survivors with these concerns may benefit if they speak to a spiritual advisor.

Physical Needs

The physical changes a cancer survivor goes through are dependent upon their cancer type and the treatment they receive. These changes can be caused by the cancer itself or the therapies used to treat the cancer. Short-term side effects occur during treatment, long-term side effects begin during treatment and continue after treatment ends, and late side effects are symptoms that appear months or years after treatment ends (6). Once treatment ends, survivors may contact their provider regarding physical changes and to confirm these changes are normal. Changes survivors may experience include:

Altered body image. Body changes, including amputations, disfigurement, and loss of organs/body parts, can impact a survivor in many ways. He or she may experience a sense of grief or loss and poor self-image, may barely recognize themselves, and may have difficulty relating to others. The inability to function from day to day, to be a sexual person, and to maintain social relationships may be linked to body image perception.

Cognitive functioning. Cancer treatment may cause problems with learning and memory. Forgetting a word, name, or thought in the middle of talking to someone is a common concern. These changes may occur during or right after treatment and are sometimes referred to as "chemo-brain." Multiple areas of consideration emerge while assessing these problems: effects of treatment, dementia, aging, distress, and depression, to name a few. Survivors often report that medical teams dismiss/minimize these symptoms even though they are a critical factor in QOL. Referral to a neuropsychologist may be needed.

Fatigue. *"Fatigue is not being tired! Cancer fatigue is when I, the survivor, can no longer experience any quality of life."*—Rita, survivor.

Fatigue is the most common side effect of cancer and its treatment and is frequently identified as a substantial barrier to QOL, no matter how much sleep a patient has had. Helping a survivor feel their best every day may include outlining exercise, diet, and stress reduction plans.

Fertility issues. Infertility can be a major source of distress for cancer survivors. Many cancer treatments can affect fertility in men and women or may make it difficult for a woman to carry a pregnancy to term. Chemotherapy, radiation to the brain or pelvic area, or pelvic surgery may all affect fertility. Some patients with cancer have the opportunity to bank sperm, eggs, embryos, or ovarian tissue before their cancer treatment begins. However, infertility treatments can be expensive, depending upon health insurance coverage.

Lymphedema. When lymph nodes are removed surgically or damaged by radiation, fluid builds up in the tissues of the arms and legs, causing swelling, pain, and limited motion. This fluid build-up can occur several months after surgery or radiation or many years later. Referral to a physical therapist may be needed.

Neuropathy. One of the most difficult treatment side effects is neuropathy, which is a tingling, burning, or numb feeling in the hands or feet attributable to nerve damage. Neuropathy can be caused by radiation, surgery, or chemotherapy. Neuropathy may improve when treatment stops or improve over time, or it may last for years. Referral to a physical therapist or neuro-oncologist may be needed.

Osteoporosis. Cancer, cancer treatment, or other side effects may cause bone loss, resulting in weaker bones that can break more easily. Referral to an endocrinologist may be needed.

Pain. Cancer pain may be short-lived or long lasting. It can be mild or severe and affect bones, nerves, and organs. Each survivor's pain will be unique—pain may be attributable to the cancer or its treatment or have nothing to do with either, and pain does not always mean that cancer has grown or returned. If a survivor experiences sudden, new pain, such as pressing chest pain, he or she should call 911 or go to the nearest emergency department. Emergency care also is recommended if a survivor has pain with fever, nausea, vomiting, or bleeding.

Sexual health. Sexuality is an integral part of human life and a quality-of-life issue. Sex fosters intimacy and shared pleasure in a relationship, and any type of cancer can negatively influence a patient's sexual health for years. When a clinician addresses sexuality issues, this indicates openness to addressing a survivor's questions and concerns. Points to consider when talking with a survivor include phases of sexual function and how cancer can affect each phase (9), factors affecting sexual function (10), and treatment options for sexual dysfunction (11,12). If further support is needed, a referral to a trained sexuality counselor for patients with cancer is recommended.

Barriers to Psychosocial Care for Cancer Survivors

Although the need for improved integration of primary medical care and behavioral healthcare is well documented, a multitude of system issues and barriers continues to negatively influence the effective delivery of psychosocial services at multiple levels. Often, knowledge is lacking regarding a patient's illness and its management, treatment goals, and influence on future health. This knowledge deficiency serves as a barrier, as does the lack of a survivor's knowledge regarding available psychosocial resources or services (1,13). Poor care coordination and treatment planning on the part of a provider (14) can also interfere with a cancer survivor's ability to access the care they need. The historical disconnect between medical care and behavioral health (1,15) is also a substantial barrier, as are inadequate or inefficient psychosocial care delivery models (16) and a lack of education regarding the importance of psychosocial services (17).

Helping Survivors Move Beyond Cancer

FEAR OF RECURRENCE
Physical changes experienced after treatment or seeing something in the media that is a reminder of somebody's cancer diagnosis can trigger a survivor's thoughts about their own cancer and the events their future may hold. Random thoughts about cancer are normal. However, if these thoughts affect QOL, a survivor may need additional coping support.

A cancer survivor's caregivers may have more fears about recurrence than the survivor. Simple strategies can help to alleviate recurrence fears for both survivors and caregivers:

■ Patients must maintain good health, keep follow-up appointments, ask questions, report symptoms, and speak freely with the medical team.
■ Patients must bear in mind that if their cancer returns, there are ways to combat it. Catching cancer early, learning about treatments, and practicing learned coping skills can go a long way toward addressing any new situations.

Empowerment Through Resilience

The cancer journey is a unique experience for everyone. Survivors often learn new skills to help with coping, adjustment, and their QOL posttreatment. Survivors are resilient and use various methods to move forward and regain normalcy in their lives. To help further empower survivors, providers should encourage patients to continue self-care, make necessary lifestyle changes, receive annual medical care, maintain a support system, reduce stress, and have fun.

Advance Care Planning and Advance Directives

Conversations with loved ones about future healthcare decisions are an essential part of advance care planning. These discussions can help survivors ensure their choices will be regarded with the utmost respect, and their family's financial and emotional burden will be lessened.

A cancer survivor may have to accept the many physical and emotional changes that can linger for years or a lifetime, including long-term treatment-related side effects, disability, or shifting treatment goals. Survivors need encouragement to engage in the process of advance care planning, which includes

- **Thinking** about what is most important to them
- **Discussing** their values, goals, and preferences for healthcare
- **Recording** this information in writing
- **Asking** their medical team and medical power of attorney to honor their wishes
- **Reviewing** this information periodically and making adjustments accordingly

Advance care planning involves five components (18)

- **Documentation**
  - The survivor's values, goals, and preferences for medical care
- **Advance directives**
  - Medical power of attorney (or durable power of attorney for healthcare)
  - Living will (or directive to physicians and families or surrogates)
  - Out-of-hospital do not resuscitate order
  - Appointment for disposition of remains
- **Financial planning**
  - Durable power of attorney (or financial power of attorney)
  - Last will and testament
  - Patients should consult an attorney regarding issues of guardianship, custody, trusts, and any special circumstances
- **Legacy planning**
  - The act of putting one's thoughts, advice, values, wishes, and so on, into actual items (e.g., a scrapbook, journal of childhood stories, or box of special mementos) the survivor's loved ones can cherish year after year
- **End-of-life planning**
  - May include consulting a spiritual advisor or prearranging funeral plans

Advance care planning professionals such as attorneys and social workers should be available to help cancer survivors and their loved ones navigate this process.

REFERENCES

1. Institute of Medicine. *Cancer Care for the Whole Patient: Meeting Psychosocial Health Needs.* Washington, DC: National Academies Press; 2008.
2. National Comprehensive Cancer Center, Fort Washington, PA. *NCCN Clinical Practice Guidelines in Oncology. Distress Management, Version 3*; 2015.
3. Philip EJ, Merluzzi TV, Zhang ZY, et al. Depression and cancer survivorship: importance of coping self-efficacy in post-treatment survivors. *Psychooncology.* 2013;22(5):987–994. doi:10.1002/pon.3088
4. Duffy JD, Valentine A. *MD Anderson Manual of Psychosocial Oncology.* New York, NY: McGraw-Hill; 2011.
5. Hewitt M, Rowland JH, Yancik R. Cancer survivors in the United States: age, health, and disability. *J Gerontol A Biol.* 2003;58(1):82–91. doi:10.1093/gerona/58.1.M82
6. The University of Texas MD Anderson Cancer Center. *Survivorship: Living with, through and beyond cancer.* Houston, TX: The University of Texas MD Anderson Cancer Center; 2012.
7. Burg MA, Adorno G, Lopez EDS, et al. Current unmet needs of cancer survivors: analysis of open-ended responses to the American Cancer Society Study of Cancer Survivors II. *Cancer.* 2015;121(4):623–630. doi:10.1002/cncr.28951
8. National Cancer Institute. Spirituality in cancer care. 2015. Available at: https://www.cancer.gov/about-cancer/coping/day-to-day/faith-and-spirituality/spirituality-pdq
9. Hughes MK. Disorders of sexuality and reproduction. In: Berger AM, Shuster JL, Von Roenn JH, eds. *Principles and Practice of Palliative Care and Supportive Oncology.* 4th ed. Philadelphia, PA: Lippincott, Williams & Wilkins; 2013.
10. Messner C, Vera T, Washington C, et al. Issues of self-image, disfigurement, and sadness in people living with cancer. *The Oncology Nurse—APN/PA.* 2013;6(3):22–26.
11. Hughes MK. Male sexuality and reproduction in patients with cancer. *inPractice.* 2016. Available at: https://www.inpractice.com/Textbooks/Oncology-Nursing/Symptom-Management/Male-Sexuality-Reproduction/Chapter-Pages/Page-1
12. Hughes MK. Female sexuality and reproduction in patients with cancer. *inPractice.* 2016. Available at: https://www.inpractice.com/Textbooks/Oncology-Nursing/Symptom-Management/Female-Sexuality-Reproduction/Chapter-Pages/Page-1.
13. Institute of Medicine. *Delivering High-Quality Cancer Care: Charting a New Course for a System in Crisis.* Washington, DC: National Academies Press; 2013.
14. Kunkel EJS, Worley LLM, Monti DA, et al. Follow-up consultation billing and documentation. *Gen Hosp Psychiatry.* 1999;21(3):197–208. doi:10.1016/S0163-8343(99)00016-X
15. Stanton E. *Integration: A 2016 Beacon Health Options White Paper.* Boston, MA: Beacon Health Strategies LLC; 2016.
16. Goldberg RJ. Financial incentives influencing the integration of mental health care and primary care. *Psych Serv.* 1999;50(8):1071–1075. doi:10.1176/ps.50.8.1071
17. Pincus HA. Depression and primary care: drowning in the mainstream or left on the banks? *J Manag Care Pharm.* 2006;12(2):S3–S9. doi:10.18553/jmcp.2006.12.S6-B.S3
18. The University of Texas MD Anderson Cancer Center. Advance care planning workbook. 2017. Available at: https://www.mdanderson.org/content/dam/mdanderson/documents/patients-and-family/becoming-our-patient/planning-for-care/Advance%20Care%20Planning%20Workbook.pdf.

5 Screening and Prevention Strategies

Therese Bevers
Suzanne Day

More patients are surviving cancer. However, an aging cancer population results in more years during which a second primary cancer (SPC) can develop.

Many cancer survivors transfer care from their oncologist to another setting, often to their primary care physician (PCP). However, many PCPs are not aware of SPC risks associated with a cancer diagnosis or treatment. This chapter provides guidance regarding SPC risk and appropriate prevention and screening interventions.

SPC ETIOLOGY

An SPC is a new primary cancer that develops in a person with a history of cancer. SPC may affect the same organ, particularly paired organs such as the breast or kidney; may occur in the same region (such as head and neck); or may arise in tissue or organs distinct from the primary cancer. Terminology is controversial; some experts do not consider contralateral breast cancer or a new colon cancer to be an SPC (1). When all SPCs are combined, SPCs are the fifth most common type of cancer after colorectal, lung, breast, and prostate cancers (2).

Overall, cancer survivors have a 14% higher risk for a new malignancy than the general population (3). SPC risk is related to longevity; cancer survivors have to live long enough to develop an SPC. Cancers associated with a lower survival rate pose lower risk for SPC because fewer patients survive long enough to develop an SPC (e.g., patients with pancreatic cancer). Sites that share a common primary carcinogenic etiology pose higher risk for SPC (e.g., survivors of head and neck cancers with a history of long-term tobacco use are at higher SPC risk for lung or other tobacco-related cancers). SPC risk varies by age and gender. Childhood cancer survivors are more likely to develop an SPC; they have an observed-to-expected ratio higher than 6 (3). This is attributable to a number of factors. Survivors of childhood cancers are more likely to have an inherited predisposition for cancer. These survivors also have many years during which to develop an SPC or age-related cancer.

Women are at slightly higher risk for SPC than men, mostly because of the higher number of female-related cancers (breast, cervix, endometrial, ovarian) than male-related cancers (testicular, prostate) (3). Risk is also higher among Black cancer survivors; the cause is not entirely understood (3).

RISK PATHWAYS

In addition to risks associated with aging, SPC may be attributable to factors associated with a primary cancer (Table 5.1). This chapter applies a systematic approach to prevention and screening strategies for SPC based on identified risks.

Genetic Risk

People with a family history of cancer in multiple relatives, especially those with early-onset cancer or other unusual presentations, may have an inherited predisposition to the disease. Genetic testing should be considered for people who have had:

- Cancer at an unusually young age (e.g., breast cancer at age 45 or younger)
- Multiple different cancers (e.g., colon and endometrial cancer in one person or breast and ovarian cancer in one family member)
- A family history involving multiple family members with a particular type of cancer or with cancers at an earlier age than expected (e.g., two or more family members with breast cancer prior to age 50)
- A family history of breast or ovarian cancer in an individual of Ashkenazi Jewish decent
- An unusual presentation of cancer (e.g., a male family member with breast cancer or a female relative with bilateral breast cancer prior to age 50)

Table 5.2 provides a list of cancers associated with selected gene mutations. People with a family history that is concerning for an inherited predisposition should be referred to a genetic counselor who is familiar with oncology risks. The National

TABLE 5.1 Pathways That Increase Risk for Primary Cancer and SPC

Risks	Areas of Concern
Genetic risks	Specific gene mutations that contribute to primary cancer risk and SPC
Lifestyle risks	Obesity Tobacco Alcohol Radiation
Biologic risks	Human papillomavirus Hepatitis C
Treatment-related risks	Radiation Hormonal Chemotherapy

SPC, second primary cancer.

Source: Bevers TB. Screening for second primary cancers. In: Foxhall LE, Rodriguez MA, eds. *Advances in Cancer Survivorship Management, MD Anderson Cancer Care Series*. Houston, TX: The University of Texas MD Anderson Cancer Center; 2014.

TABLE 5.2 Genetic Mutations That Increase Risk for Multiple Cancers

Gene Mutation	Cancer Risks
BRCA mutations	Breast Ovarian Prostate Pancreas
Lynch syndrome	Colon, small intestine, stomach, bile duct Kidney, ureter Ovary, endometrium Brain

Li Fraumeni syndrome	Core cancers
	    Soft-tissue sarcoma and osteosarcoma
	    Breast (premenopausal)
	    Adrenocortical carcinoma
	    Brain tumors
	Other cancers
	    Hypodiploid acute lymphoblastic
	      leukemias
	    Melanoma

Cowden syndrome	Breast Thyroid Endometrial Colorectal Renal Melanoma

Source: National Comprehensive Cancer Network. The NCCN Screening and Diagnosis Guidelines in Oncology (Version 1.2016). Available at: http://www.nccn.org

Society of Genetic Counselors provides cancer risk genetic testing guidance and a position statement on the use of multigene panels and is a genetic counselor locator resource (4).

Lifestyle Factors

Lifestyle and environmental factors that contributed to a primary cancer may influence development of an SPC.

TOBACCO

Tobacco use poses increased risk for cancers of the lung, esophagus, larynx, pharynx, oral cavity, cervix, kidney, bladder, and pancreas. Smokeless tobacco use increases oral cavity cancer risk. There is a synergistic effect between alcohol and tobacco use, resulting in a higher cancer risk with the use of both as opposed to the use of one alone.

ALCOHOL

Alcohol use is associated with a convincing increased risk for cancers of the oral cavity (mouth and pharynx), larynx and esophagus, and colon (men only). Probable increased risk exists for liver cancer and colorectal cancer (women) (5).

Convincing increased risk is associated with alcohol use and breast cancer. When compared with nondrinkers, women who consume approximately 0.5 to 1 drink per day have a relative risk (RR) of 1.03. Those who consume 1.5 to 2 drinks per day have an RR of 1.13, 2.5 to 3 drinks per day increases RR to 1.21, and 3.5 to 4 drinks per day increases RR to 1.32 (breast cancer RR increases by approximately 7% per 10 g of alcohol consumed per day). Results are consistent in multiple epidemiology studies. In developed countries, 4% of breast cancer may be attributed to alcohol consumption. Alcohol type does not influence risk (6).

OBESITY

Obesity is associated with convincing increased risk for postmenopausal breast cancer and cancers of the colon, endometrium, esophagus, kidney, and pancreas. Obesity also may increase risk for cancers of the gallbladder (probable increased risk) and liver (limited suggestion of risk) (7).

Biologic/Viral Risks

Human papillomavirus (HPV), a risk factor for cervical, vaginal, vulvar, anal, penile, and oropharyngeal cancers, is the sole contemporary cause of cervical cancer. It is the leading cause of anal and penile cancers and is overtaking tobacco use as the cause of cancers of the oropharynx. HPV strains 16 and 18 pose the highest risk for cancer; 70% of all cervical and oropharyngeal cancers are caused by HPV 16 or 18. HPV strains 31, 33, 35, 39, 45, 51, 52, 56, 58, 59, and 68 also increase cancer risk (8).

Treatment-Related Risks

Chemotherapy, radiation therapy, and serial imaging increase risk for SPC. Cancer survivors who have received chemotherapy are at higher risk for leukemia than the general population. Iatrogenic exposure to ionizing radiation increases risk for skin cancers, sarcomas, and cancers of the organs within the radiation field (9). Breast cancer risk is 3-fold higher following mantle/thoracic radiation in young women with Hodgkin's lymphoma who are treated during the second and third decades of life (10).

Selective estrogen receptor modulators increase risk for endometrial cancer when used in breast cancer survivors or women at increased risk for breast cancer. Although risk is increased, studies have not demonstrated a benefit for endometrial cancer screening.

Other therapeutic variables influence cancer risk. Multiple ionizing imaging studies conducted over time contribute to cancer risk. In addition, some people are particularly susceptible to ionizing radiation, typically because of a genetic predisposition. For example, risk for cancer, particularly sarcomas, is increased among people with Li-Fraumeni syndrome.

It is important to understand and clearly communicate to survivors that treatment-related SPCs are attributable to the successful treatment of their primary cancer. Had they not survived the original cancer, they would not be at risk for this SPC.

RISK REDUCTION

Lifestyle/Environmental

Reducing cancer risk entails removing risk-provoking agents or behaviors from a patient's environment or removing the patient from a risk-laden environment. A healthy lifestyle must be encouraged for all survivors to improve their overall health and quality of life and reduce risk for disease and death. Fortunately, survivors are highly motivated people. Clinicians must capitalize on each teachable moment even if a negative behavior did not contribute to a primary cancer. It is important to bear in mind that improving a survivor's overall health can also positively influence the health of the survivor's caregivers and family. If a patient needs community support to assist with long-term abstinence or behavior changes, be sure to provide proven resources.

TOBACCO
All patients must be assessed for tobacco use. Follow these guidelines (11):

- **Ask** if the patient is using tobacco products
- **Assess** attitudes toward tobacco use and quitting the habit
- **Advise** regarding cessation
- **Assist** with the cessation plan
- **Arrange** cessation follow-up

Cessation is an ongoing process, so reassess at regular intervals and restart the process if relapse occurs.

Medications that reduce the desire for nicotine include (12):

- Varenicline (Chantix), which blocks nicotine effects and reduces cravings and withdrawal symptoms; smokers experience decreased satisfaction with tobacco use
- Bupropion (Zyban), an antidepressant, which reduces withdrawal symptoms
- Alternative tobacco delivery systems such as patches, nicotine gum, lozenges, and inhalers, which gradually reduce nicotine levels

ALCOHOL
Alcohol consumption should be limited for survivors who choose to drink. Women should consume no more than one drink per day and men no more than two drinks per day. One drink is equivalent to 12 ounces of beer, 5 ounces of wine, or 1.5 ounces of hard liquor (13). Clinicians should assist with alcohol addiction/abuse scenarios by providing psychosocial support, medications, and methods to reduce symptoms of withdrawal and prevent relapse. Comorbid conditions including anxiety, depression, and bipolar disease should also be treated (11).

ENERGY BALANCE

The American Institute for Cancer Research (AICR), which is an international network dedicated to cancer prevention, provides evidence-based healthy lifestyle recommendations for people without cancer and cancer survivors (Table 5.3). According to the AICR, cancer survivors should follow the same cancer prevention guidelines as people who have not had cancer.

Survivors should strive to achieve and maintain a healthy body weight through energy balance (calories consumed [diet] vs. calories expended [physical activity]). The target body mass index (BMI) score is 18.5 to 24.9. BMI scores between 25.0 and 29.9 denote being overweight, and a BMI score of 30 or higher denotes obesity. AICR recommendations include maintaining a lean BMI score between 21 and 23 (this is a more narrow BMI range than that established by other agencies) and maintaining a healthy weight over the life span (13).

Physical activity is encouraged. Survivors should be prompted to participate in 150 minutes of moderate activity (able to talk, but not sing) per week or 75 minutes of vigorous activity (they can say a few words but not full sentences) per week. Strength training should be done twice a week (14). The most important clinical message is that sedentary activity should be limited.

AICR has specific dietary recommendations, advocating for limited consumption of energy-dense food and drinks. This means sparingly consuming high-calorie foods (food with >225–275 calories per 100 g), avoiding sugary drinks, limiting fruit juice, and avoiding or limiting "fast food" and convenience foods, which tend to be high in calories and fat (13).

AICR also recommends a plant-based diet that calls for at least five daily servings of nonstarchy vegetables and fruits and unprocessed grains and legumes at every meal. AICR encourages patients to consume less than 500 g of red meat per week and avoid or limit processed meats. Patients also should avoid salt-preserved and salty foods (limit to 2.4 g sodium per day) and moldy grains/legumes. As previously noted,

TABLE 5.3 American Institute for Cancer Research Guidelines

Cancer Survivors Should Follow the Same Cancer Prevention Guidelines as People Who Have Not Had Cancer

- Maintain a lean body mass index between 21 and 23
- Be physically active
- Limit consumption of energy-dense food and drinks
- Eat mostly plant-based foods
- Limit intake of red meat and avoid processed meats
- Limit alcohol to 1 drink per day for women and 2 drinks per day for men
- Avoid salt-preserved and salty foods and moldy grains/legumes
- Discuss supplements with a provider before taking them
- Breastfeed infants for 6 months, if possible

Source: World Cancer Research Fund/American Institute for Cancer Research. *Food, Nutrition, Physical Activity, and the Prevention of Cancer: A Global Perspective*. Washington, DC: American Institute for Cancer Research, 2007.

alcohol should be limited to one drink per day for women and two drinks per day for men. Processed foods with salt added should be limited. Patients should discuss supplements with their provider before taking them; optimally, they should avoid supplements and achieve nutritional goals through food intake (13). New mothers should breastfeed their infants for 6 months if possible.

SUN EXPOSURE

SPF 30 or higher sunscreen with ultraviolet A and B protection should be used to ensure adequate coverage. Sunscreen should be applied 30 minutes before sun exposure and reapplied frequently, particularly after swimming or sweating (15). Sun exposure during peak sun hours and tanning beds should be avoided.

VACCINES

The HPV vaccine is approved for males and females ages 9 to 26. The target population for the HPV vaccine is boys and girls between 11 and 12 years of age. Children may receive the vaccine as early as age 9, and there is a catch-up period between 13 and 26 years of age. Two doses are required for children ages 9 to 14, and 3 doses are required for people ages 15 to 26 (16).

There are three types of HPV vaccine. The bivalent vaccine is effective for HPV 16 and 18. The quadrivalent vaccine is effective for HPV 6, 11, 16, and 18. HPV 6 and 11 cause 90% of all genital warts. HPV 16 and 18 cause 70% of cervical and oropharyngeal cancers. The 9-valent vaccine is effective for HPV 6, 11, 16, 18, 31, 33, 45, 52, and 58. The 9-valent vaccine is estimated to reduce risk for HPV-related cancers by 90%. If the bivalent or quadrivalent vaccine has previously been administered, patients do not need to be revaccinated with the 9-valent vaccine. If used effectively, the vaccine could eliminate more than 30,000 HPV-related cancers each year in United States.

Despite their availability and endorsement by the Centers for Disease Control and Prevention and the National Cancer Institute, these vaccines are underused. Only 41.9% of girls and 28.1% of boys have completed the prescribed series of vaccinations.

Breast Cancer Risk Reduction Therapy

Risk assessment using the Breast Cancer Risk Assessment Tool or "Gail Model" can help to identify at-risk women ages 35 and older who may be candidates for risk reduction therapy. Patients are considered to be at increased risk for breast cancer if their 5-year risk is 1.7% or higher. The Tyrer-Cuzick model is another computerized tool that can be used to estimate breast cancer risk based on a more extensive family history. Increased risk is considered to be a 10-year risk of 5% or higher. Lifetime breast cancer risk of 20% or higher according to either model is considered increased risk. Women with a history of lobular carcinoma in situ (LCIS), atypical ductal hyperplasia, or atypical lobular hyperplasia are considered to be at high breast cancer risk, as are women who received thoracic radiation between ages 10 and 30.

Women with a 5-year breast cancer risk of 1.7% or higher according to the Gail Model or 10-year breast cancer risk of 5% or higher according to the Tyrer-Cuzick model may be candidates for risk reduction therapy after assessing the balance of benefits and harms. Tamoxifen 20 mg daily for 5 years is the only agent approved for use in at-risk premenopausal women. At-risk postmenopausal women are candidates for 5 years of preventive therapy with tamoxifen 20 mg daily, raloxifene 60 mg daily, or an aromatase inhibitor (exemestane 25 mg daily or anastrozole 1 mg daily) (11,12). Of note, aromatase inhibitors are not currently Food and Drug Administration (FDA) approved for breast cancer risk reduction.

Therapy benefit is most notable for women with high-risk proliferative breast lesions (atypical [ductal, lobular] hyperplasia or LCIS). In the absence of an absolute contraindication such as a venous thromboembolic event history, these women should be strongly considered for risk reduction therapy (12). Risk reduction therapy is not indicated for women with a life expectancy of less than 10 years or contraindications to therapy. Use prior to age 35 has not been investigated and is dependent on competing risks such as breast cancer risk versus planned pregnancies.

A nonstatistically significant reduction in breast cancer risk has been noted for women with a BRCA2 mutation, but not women with a BRCA1 mutation (17).This finding is concordant with clinical findings of BRCA2 mutation carriers being more likely to develop a hormonally sensitive breast cancer, whereas BRCA1 mutation carriers are more likely to have hormone-negative breast cancer. Tamoxifen can reduce risk for hormone-sensitive breast cancers but not hormone-negative breast cancers.

Prophylactic Surgery

People with genetic predispositions are at very high risk for cancer. In certain situations, prophylactic surgery can substantially reduce cancer risk. Bilateral prophylactic mastectomy (BPM) and risk-reducing salpingo-oophorectomy (RRSO) are options for women with a BRCA mutation that places them at high risk for breast and ovarian cancers (11). Individuals with familial adenomatous polyposis are at extremely high risk for colon cancer; they are candidates for prophylactic colectomy (11).

SPC SCREENING

Routine cancer screening for individuals with or without cancer should be based on age- and gender-specific risks related to common cancers such as breast, cervical, prostate, and colorectal cancers. However, cancer survivors face unique risks and may need additional screening. MD Anderson has developed a series of cancer screening algorithms that outline recommendations for people at average and increased risk for a first cancer or SPC (11). These algorithms are updated annually, incorporating the latest data on screening strategies, including those for cancer survivors.

Some clinical scenarios warrant consideration for supplemental screening for SPC in cancer survivors:

■ Current or former (quit within the last 15 years) smokers with a 30-plus pack-year smoking history and age between 55 and 80 should be considered for lung cancer screening

- Women who received mantle radiation between ages 10 and 30 are at high risk for breast cancer and should obtain high-risk screening with breast MRI.
- Women with a BRCA mutation are at high risk for breast cancer. Women who have not had BPM should obtain high-risk screening with breast MRI
- Women with a BRCA mutation are at increased risk for ovarian cancer. Women who have not had RRSO should obtain high-risk screening for ovarian cancer
- Women with Lynch syndrome are at increased risk for endometrial cancer and should consider prophylactic hysterectomy with or without removal of ovaries. If prophylactic surgery is not performed, endometrial cancer screening is recommended

Although individuals with HPV are at risk for a number of cancers, there are currently no screening recommendations other than screening for cervical cancer. Nonetheless, patients and partners should be counseled regarding risk at other sites (cervical, vaginal, vulvar, anal, penile, oral) and encouraged to monitor for any changes.

Every survivorship visit should include an assessment of SPC risks, risk reduction strategies, and appropriate screenings.

REFERENCES

1. Krueger H, McLean D, Williams D. *The Prevention of Second Primary Cancers. Progress in Experimental Tumor Research.* Vol 40. New York, NY: Basek Karger; 2008.
2. Rheingold SR, Neugut AL, Medows AT. Secondary cancers: incidence, risk factors, and management. In: Bast RC, Kufe DW, Pollock RE, et al, eds. *Cancer Medicine.* Hamilton, Ontario: BC Decker; 2000.
3. Fraumeni JF Jr, Curtis RE, Edwards BK, et al. Introduction. In: Curtis RE, Freedman DM, Ron E, et al, eds. *New Malignancies Among Cancer Survivors: SEER Cancer Registries, 1973–2000.* NIH Pub No. 05-5302. Bethesda, MD: National Cancer Institute; 2006.
4. National Society of Genetic Counselors. Position statement on the use of multi-gene panel tests. March 14, 2017. Available at www.nscg.org
5. World Cancer Research Fund/American Institute for Cancer Research. *Food, Nutrition, Physical Activity, and the Prevention of Cancer: A Global Perspective.* Washington, DC: American Institute for Cancer Research, 2007.
6. Beral V, Hamajima N, Hirose K, et al. Alcohol, tobacco and breast cancer—collaborative reanalysis of individual data from 53 epidemiological studies, including 58515 women with breast cancer and 95067 women without the disease. *Br J Cancer.* 2002;87(11):1234–1245.
7. Lauby-Secretan B, Scoccianti C, Loomis D, et al. Body fatness and cancer–viewpoint of the IARC Working Group. *N Engl J Med.* 2016;375(8):794–798.
8. Saslow D, Solomon D, Lawson HW, et al. American Cancer Society, American Society for Colposcopy and Cervical Pathology, and American Society for Clinical Pathology. Screening guidelines for the prevention and early detection of cervical cancer. *Am J Clin Pathol.* 2012;137:516–542.
9. Bevers TB. Screening for second primary cancers. In: Foxhall LE, Rodriguez MA, eds. *Advances in Cancer Survivorship Management, MD Anderson Cancer Care Series.* Houston, TX: The University of Texas MD Anderson Cancer Center; 2014.

10. Travis LB, Hill D, Dores GM, et al. Breast cancer following radiotherapy and chemotherapy among young women with Hodgkin's disease. *JAMA*. 2003;290:465–475.

11. National Comprehensive Cancer Network. The NCCN Screening and Diagnosis Guidelines in Oncology (Version 1.2016). Available at: http://www.nccn.org

12. The University of Texas MD Anderson Cancer Center. *Cancer screening and risk reduction algorithms*. Available at www.mdanderson.org

13. American Institute for Cancer Research (AICR), World Cancer Research Fund International (WCRF). *Food, Nutrition, Physical Activity, and the Prevention of Cancer: A Global Perspective*. Washington, DC: AICR/WCRF; 2007.

14. American College of Sports Medicine, Irwin ML. ACSM's Guide to Exercise and Cancer Survivorship. Champaign, IL: Human Kinetics; 2012.

15. American Academy of Dermatology. Position statement on broad spectrum protection of sunscreen products. November 14, 2009. Available at: www.aad.org

16. Meites E, Kempe A, Markowitz LE. Use of a 2-dose schedule for human papillomavirus vaccination–updated recommendations of the Advisory Committee on Immunization Practices. *MMWR*. 2016;65(49):1405–1408.

17. King MC, Weiand S, Hale K, et al. Tamoxifen and breast cancer incidence among women with inherited mutations in BRCA1 and BRCA2: National Surgical Adjuvant Breast and Bowel Project (NSABP) breast cancer prevention trial. *JAMA*. 2001;286:2251–2256.

6 The Older Adult Cancer Survivor

Beatrice J. Edwards
Linda Pang
Maria Suarez Almazor

The worldwide population is aging as life spans extend and the birth rate declines. The result is that European countries now have the oldest populations in the world. This demographic change affects oncology practice; currently, 60% of patients with cancer are 65 years of age and older, and this will increase to 70% by 2030. Cancer survivor numbers are on the rise, with 14.5 million survivors in 2014 and an expected 19 million by 2024 (1).

Life expectancy should be the first priority when determining treatment choices. Life expectancy at age "X" is defined as the average number of years remaining to be lived by a member of a survivorship group who is exactly age "X." The ePrognosis tool (eprognosis.ucsf.edu) is one with which life expectancy may be calculated. Most life expectancy estimates involve use of current life tables, meaning that age-specific mortality experiences of the current population are used.

Failure to consider prognosis in the context of clinical decision making can lead to poor care. For example, healthy older patients with a good prognosis experience low rates of cancer screening. But older adults with advanced dementia or metastatic cancer often are screened for slow-growing cancers that are unlikely to cause symptoms. Such screenings, however, may lead to distress resulting from false-positive results, invasive workups, and treatments. In recognition of these issues, guidelines increasingly incorporate life expectancy as a central factor in weighing the benefits and the burdens of tests and treatments.

One systematic review (2) identified prognostic indicators. Predictors for community-dwelling older adults include the Gagne 12-month predictor, which has been validated in a nationally representative sample. The Yourman et al. index for prediction of 5-year mortality was developed from the 1997 to 2000 National Health Interview Survey, which was well calibrated and had good discrimination in a random sample of 8,038 adults drawn from the same data source (2). This index is of particular relevance when screening older adults.

GERIATRIC ONCOLOGY ASSESSMENT

Geriatric oncology usually refers to a specialty that cares for older adults (65 years of age and older) with cancer. Geriatric assessment extends beyond the traditional disease-oriented medical evaluation of an older person's health; included are assessments of cognitive, affective, functional, social, economic, environmental, and spiritual status as well as a discussion of patient preferences regarding advance directives (Figure 6.1). This approach recognizes that the health status of older people is dependent upon influences beyond the manifestations of their medical conditions such as social, psychological, and environmental factors. Geriatric assessment also places high value on functional status, both as a dimension to be evaluated and as an outcome to be improved or maintained. Although in the strictest sense *geriatric assessment* is a diagnostic process, many use the term to include both evaluation and management (3). Geriatric assessments may be performed in outpatient and inpatient settings that include inpatient rehabilitation facilities and geriatric evaluation units at veterans hospitals; assessment models such as Geriatric Resources for Assessment and Care of Elders and Guided Care of the Elderly specialty programs may be used (3).

Geriatric assessment is a systematic procedure used to appraise objective health, including multimorbidity and functional status that can interfere with cancer prognosis and treatment choices in older cancer patients (Table 6.1) (4). Usefulness of Comprehensive Geriatric Assessment (CGA) has been well summarized by Wildiers et al (4). It is useful for:

1. Revealing undiagnosed conditions that are not found during routine oncology care.
2. Predicting toxicity/adverse effects from cancer treatment or a decrease in quality of life (QOL), enabling more targeted use of preventive measures.
3. Obtaining important prognostic information about life expectancy that is of paramount importance when making treatment decisions.
4. Geriatric assessment that can influence/improve treatment decisions.
5. Targeted interventions that can improve QOL and compliance.

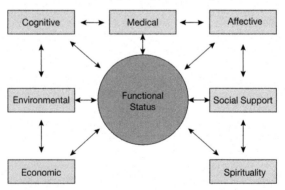

FIGURE 6.1 Comprehensive Geriatric Assessment domains.
Sources: From Fagard K, Leonard S, Deschodt M, et al. The impact of frailty on postoperative outcomes in individuals aged 65 and over undergoing elective surgery for colorectal cancer: a systematic review. *J Geriatr Oncol*. 2016;7(6):479–491; Lord S. Falls. In: Halter JB, Ouslander JG, Studenski S, et al, eds. *Hazzard's Geriatric Medicine and Gerontology*. New York, NY: McGraw Hill Education; 2016:723–732; Reuben DB, Rosen S, Schickedanz HB. Principles of geriatric assessment. In: Halter JB, Studenski S, High KP, et al., eds. *Hazzard's Geriatric Medicine and Gerontology*. 7th ed. *(Kindle Location 7621)*. New York, NY: McGraw-Hill Education; 2016:157–171.

TABLE 6.1 Geriatric Assessment Components

Scales	Thresholds for Diagnosis	Diagnosis
Bone health	BMD T-score range between −1.0 and −2.5 SD	Osteopenia (low bone mass)
	BMD T-score < −2.5 SD	Osteoporosis
Comorbidity	Charlson Comorbidity Index score > 4.0	Comorbidity
Neurocognitive testing	MoCA rapid screening instrument for mild cognitive dysfunction	Mild cognitive dysfunction
	MoCA score > 26 or above is normal (maximum = 30)	Normal
	Parental history of dementia, concussions, strokes, hypertension, diabetes, hyperlipidemia, cognitive impairment for several months or years (not an acute condition)	
	MoCA score < 26	Mild cognitive dysfunction
	If IADLs are intact	Mild cognitive impairment
	Impairment in at least two IADLs (finances, taking own medications, using the telephone, transportation, shopping) and abnormal MoCA score	Dementia
	If using the Mini-Cog test, abnormalities in 3-item recall or clock drawing	Referral for cognitive testing needed
Malnutrition	Mini Nutritional Assessment	
	Score 12–14	Normal
	Score 8–11	At risk for malnutrition
	Score 0–7	Malnourished
Gait disorders	Short Physical Performance Battery	
	Score 10–12	Normal
	Score ≤ 9	Balance and gait disorder
Frailty (37)	Fried criteria: Low hand-grip strength <20 kg (F) and <30 kg (M)	3 criteria present denotes frailty
	Slow gait (<1.0 m/s), exhaustion ("yes" answers to two questions: "everything I do requires an effort" and "I could not get going"), weight loss, sedentary lifestyle	
Functional ADLs	Katz: ADLs 6 items: bathing, toileting, grooming, feeding, transfers, and continence Normal score: 6	Functional impairment ADL score < 5

(continued)

TABLE 6.1 Geriatric Assessment Components *(continued)*

Scales	Thresholds for Diagnosis	Diagnosis
Independent IADLs	Lawton-Brody: Managing finances, taking own medications, using the telephone, able to travel independently, and shopping Score 5	Absence of two IADLs necessary for dementia diagnosis
Depression	Patient Health Questionnaire-9 Score > 10	88% sensitivity, 88% specificity for major depression
Polypharmacy	More than four medications Beers criteria	
Social support	Multiple Outcomes Study	<75% = poor social support

ADL, activities of daily living; BMD, bone mineral density; IADL, instrumental activities of daily living; MoCA, Montreal Cognitive Assessment; SD, standard deviation.

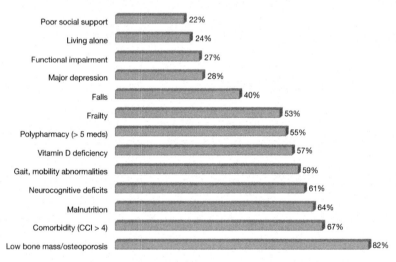

FIGURE 6.2 Functional and social status and medical diagnoses identified through Comprehensive Geriatric Assessment.
CCI, Charlson Comorbidity Index.

Studies have described a number of new diagnoses that are identified during cancer care in older patients. As a result, care of older cancer survivors should focus on managing comorbidities and late effects of cancer care and awareness of possible underlying geriatric conditions (Figure 6.2). Managing such conditions is important because studies in noncancer populations reveal that such geriatric syndromes are associated with adverse outcomes including increased hospitalization rates and overall mortality. Also, a patient may present with several new diagnoses, and interventions may need to be initiated more than once.

For example, a 75-year-old man who is a lung cancer survivor is seen for survivorship services. He has lost 10 pounds during the last 6 months, is experiencing falls, and has anorexia. He will need an evaluation for cancer recurrence, a nutritional consultation and intervention, and a protein-calorie-dense diet. Clinicians also need to determine if his anorexia is related to depression. If depression is confirmed, this patient will receive antidepressants and orexigenic agents (e.g., mirtazapine or megestrol). He will be referred to physical therapy for gait and balance training and be tested for vitamin D level. Because low bone mass and fractures are common among older patients with cancer, calcium and vitamin D supplementation and a bone density test will be recommended. If a bone density test reveals low bone mass (osteopenia) or osteoporosis, this patient also should receive an FDA-approved medication for osteoporosis (Tables 6.2 and 6.3).

TABLE 6.2 Targeted Geriatric Interventions

Domains	Geriatric Interventions
Cognitive	Evaluate for reversible factors for memory loss Brain imaging (CT/MRI brain) Therapeutic trial of acetyl cholinesterase inhibitors or cognitive enhancers Speech therapy for cognitive training Exercise (improves mild cognitive impairment)
Bone health	Calcium and vitamin D recommendations Exercise recommendations Use of antiresorptive medications
Gait and balance disorders	Assess and replace vitamin D (in insufficiency or deficiency) Physical therapy for gait and balance training
Falls	Strength training Tai chi Home safety evaluation
Polypharmacy	Eliminate adverse medications (Beers criteria) Reduce the number of medicines Avoid drug-drug interactions
Malnutrition	Nutrition consultation Nutritional intervention (high-protein, high-calcium diet) Use of orexigenic agents
Frailty	Nutritional intervention and physical therapy Exercise
Sensory impairment	Use of hearing aids Use of glasses
Living alone or poor	Social work consultation
Social support	Community resources Case management for rehabilitation Home aide through the Division on Aging Adult protective services
Karnofsky scale	Physical and occupational therapy Nutrition consult Nutritional intervention

TABLE 6.3 Risk Factors for Falls (40)

Intrinsic factors

Lower extremity weakness

Poor grip strength

Balance disorders

Functional and cognitive impairment

Visual deficits

History of falls

Gait deficit

Urinary incontinence

Chronic disease

Extrinsic factors

Polypharmacy

Environmental

Poor lighting

Loose carpets

Poor access to healthcare

Low income and education levels

FRAILTY'S IMPLICATIONS IN CANCER CARE

Frailty is the state of decreased reserve and resistance to physical and emotional stressors caused by a continuous decline in various organ functions. Frailty is more common among elderly people. Patients with cancer tend to be more frail than those who remain cancer free (5), and cancer treatments may result in frailty (6).

Frailty is an important predictor of serious adverse events such as disability, poor clinical outcomes and healthcare utilization, and death (7). The frailty phenotype includes these characteristics: unintentional weight loss, weakness, slow gait, exhaustion, and low activity. In addition, there is a complex relationship between frailty and cognitive functioning (8). Three of the five frailty characteristics must be present to confirm a frailty diagnosis. In the cancer setting, frailty is associated with a guarded prognosis and a higher likelihood of chemotherapy toxicity. In survivorship care, similar risks for adverse outcomes are present.

Cancer care may contribute to frailty, chemotherapy-associated anorexia, and weight loss, all of which can lead to malnutrition. Muscle loss that is characteristic of aging is accentuated by immobility, which contributes to sarcopenia. Clinicians who provide care to cancer survivors must be attuned to this condition, which is amenable to interventions. Nutritional supplementation and exercise also are effective against frailty.

POLYPHARMACY

To prescribe appropriately, clinicians should consider age-related physiologic changes and comorbidities including cognitive impairment, functional difficulties, and caregiver issues. Older adults are at higher risk for toxicity because of diminished physiologic reserve and changes in pharmacokinetics and pharmacodynamics (Table 6.4) (9).

Principles of prescribing for older adults include starting with a low dose and titrating slowly upward. Clinicians should avoid initiating two medications at the same time. To reduce polypharmacy, prior to starting a new medication, consider its necessity and determine if there are nonpharmacologic ways to treat the condition. Consider methods with which to assess for therapeutic end points. If a medication's benefits potentially outweigh the risks, also consider the potential for drug–drug or drug–disease interactions. For older adults, there may be a medication cascade in which one medication is being used to treat the adverse effect of another, and it is important for providers to be aware of this issue (10). It is best to simplify the medication regimen, so consider if one medication can be used to address two conditions.

TABLE 6.4 Age-Associated Changes in Pharmacokinetics and Pharmacodynamics

Parameter	Age Effect	Prescribing Implications
Absorption	Rate and extent are usually unaffected	Drug-drug and drug-food interactions are more likely to alter absorption
Distribution	Increase in fat:water ratio; decreased plasma protein, particularly albumin	Fat-soluble drugs have a larger volume of distribution; highly protein-bound drugs have a greater (active) free concentration
Metabolism	Decreases in liver mass and liver blood flow decrease drug clearance; may be age-related changes in CYP2C19 whereas CYP3A4 and CYP2D6 are not affected	Lower dosages may be therapeutic
Elimination	Primarily renal; age-related decrease in glomerular filtration rate	Serum creatinine not a reliable measure of kidney function
Pharmacody-namics	Less predictable and often altered drug response at usual or lower concentrations	Prolonged pain relief with opioids at lower dosages; increased sedation and postural instability with benzodiazepines; altered sensitivity to beta blockers

Source: From Park J, Hughes AK. Nonpharmacological approaches to the management of chronic pain in community-dwelling older adults: a review of empirical evidence. *J Am Geriatr Soc.* 2012;60(3):555–568. By permission from John Wiley and Sons.

At least annually, ask the patient to bring all medications including prescription, over-the-counter, supplements, and herbal preparations to the office for review and ask about medication-related adverse events. The American Geriatrics Society Beers Criteria are an evidence-based source with which clinicians can identify potentially inappropriate medication use. Recommendations cover five categories: drugs to avoid, drugs to avoid in patients with specific diseases or syndromes, drugs to use with caution, selected drugs for which dose should be adjusted based on kidney function, and selected drug–drug interactions that are associated with harmful outcomes in older adults.

FALLS

Falls are a serious problem among older patients who have had cancer (11). Approximately one in 10 falls is injurious with consequences such as hip fracture, subdural hematoma, and traumatic brain injury (12). Falls are the most common cause of accidental death for those 75 years of age and older. Other fall-related consequences include fear of falling, impaired mobility, functional dependence, and need for institutional care (13). About 37% to 56% of all falls lead to minor injuries, and 10% to 15% of falls cause major injuries. Falls are the leading cause of injury-related hospitalizations in people ages 65 and older and account for 14% of emergency admissions and 4% of all hospital admissions in this age group (13). Older adults undergoing cancer care are at elevated risk for falls because aging-related changes may be accentuated by the effects of cancer and cancer therapy. Sarcopenia is an example; age-related muscle loss will be accelerated by cancer care treatments such as chemotherapy and corticosteroid use (14,15).

As a result of age-related changes, disease, or adverse medication effects, sensorimotor and balance systems may become impaired and predispose people to falls. Numerous variables play a role in fall occurrence: medical conditions (stroke, Parkinson's disease, dementia), medications (especially psychoactive medications), taking more than four medications, psychosocial factors (depression, female gender), functional impairment, sensorimotor function, muscle weakness, impaired balance or vision, and environmental conditions (poor footwear and external hazards) (13,16).

Sarcopenia can lead to falls and adverse clinical outcomes (17). Falls have been well described in older adult populations, yet few studies have addressed falls among older patients undergoing cancer care. Cancer is a disease of aging, so as the population continues to age, cancer incidence will increase. When assessing an older person, inquire about falls during the previous 6 months; these falls are predictive of new falls. Balance and gait assessments can include the get-up-and-go test, the 6-minute walk test, or the Short Physical Performance Battery. Individuals at risk for falls will benefit from physical therapy, evaluation of vitamin D level, and exercise. Bone health also should be evaluated in people at fall risk.

MALNUTRITION

Malnutrition in older adults leads to elevated mortality rates (18,19), reduced QOL (20,21), and functional decline (22). Malnutrition also is a major risk factor for adverse outcomes such as poor treatment response (23), chemotherapy-related toxicity (24–26), infection (27), and longer hospital stays (28–30).

Malnutrition is common among cancer patients, with prevalence ranging from 30% to 85% (31). Patients with gastrointestinal and head and neck cancers are most susceptible to malnutrition (32). However, patients with cancer are among the most malnourished yet underdiagnosed patient groups (33,34). Cancer-associated malnutrition is multifactorial; causes include local tumor effects, host response to the tumor, and effects of anticancer therapies (25). Nutritional assessment and screening tools can help to identify malnutrition status among patients with cancer.

Common malnutrition screening tools used with older adults include the Mini Nutritional Assessment and tools available from the American Society for Parenteral and Enteral Nutrition. Nutritional interventions often are necessary, including recommendations for a high-protein diet, nutrition consult, and proper hydration.

BALANCE AND GAIT REHABILITATION

Rehabilitation is a valuable component of cancer survivorship programs. Balance, the ability to maintain the center of gravity over the base of support within a given sensory environment, involves several subcomponents and is influenced by several systems. Human balance is a complex neuromusculoskeletal process involving sensory detection of body motions, integration of sensorimotor information within the central nervous system (CNS), and programming and execution of appropriate neuromuscular responses. The brain uses visual, vestibular, and somatosensory systems to determine body position and movement in space. Although there are age-related changes in these systems, older adults who are standing or walking do not display increased postural sway when compared with younger adults when all three subcomponents are available. Information from the various sensory systems is relayed to the CNS and is integrated in several areas including the vestibular nuclei and the cerebellum prior to the generation of appropriate motor responses.

When assessing an older adult, the most important area that necessitates assessment is risk for falling. Numerous fall screening tools are well validated, including the Short Physical Performance Battery, the get-up-and-go test, and the Falls Efficacy Scale, among others (35).

Treatment of balance disorders is based on specific impairments (e.g., range of motion, strength, decreased sensation, pain, use of sensory inputs, and motor strategies) and functional limitations identified during an evaluation. Balance strategies and the ability to use sensory information for balance can be learned with appropriate exercise and practice. For balance training, it is important to provide opportunities for patients to practice tasks that allow them to use the necessary balance strategies and, when possible, to incorporate the tasks into functional activities. The American Geriatrics Society/British Geriatrics Society Panel for Prevention of Falls recommends multicomponent exercises including strength, balance coordination, and gait training. Their research review indicates benefits can be obtained in programs lasting longer than 12 weeks with participation one to three times weekly (36).

Randomized clinical trials have demonstrated that exercise improves balance in community-dwelling older adults (37,38). A systematic review with a meta-analysis of 44 randomized controlled trials with a total of 9,603 subjects assess the effectiveness of exercise for fall preventions in older community and residential care adults (39). The pooled effect of 44 trials revealed a 17% reduction in falls, and importantly, the benefits were more pronounced among people who exercised for more than 50 hours in the intervention program (39). This 50-hour threshold is more effective against fall reduction if it is achieved within 6 months as opposed to 12 months (39).

Successful exercise interventions need to be custom designed and sustained for more than 12 weeks. The optimal fall prevention exercise type, duration, and intensity is a topic of debate. Exercise may be more effective for fall prevention, however, when it is combined with interventions such as home modifications and education (35,36).

SCREENING FOR SECONDARY CANCERS

Most patients with cancer are older adults, and this trend will continue to increase. Clinicians must become familiar with age-related changes and the ways in which cancer screening can benefit this population. Table 6.5 features cancer recurrence screening recommendations. Geriatric assessment is an invaluable tool in this regard and allows clinicians to develop targeted interventions to help seniors maintain functional independence and the highest possible QOL.

TABLE 6.5 Screening for Cancer Recurrence in Patients at Standard Risk

Cancer Type	Recommendations
Breast	Mammogram yearly
Prostate	Prostate-specific antigen, digital rectal exam
Lung	Chest CT
Colorectal	Chest/abdominal/pelvic CT every 3–5 years, carcinoembryonic antigen test every 6 months until 6 years, rectosigmoidoscopy every 6–12 months for 3–5 years
Bladder	Chest/abdominal/pelvic CT, urine cytology, liver functions, creatinine clearance for up to 2 years
Thyroid	Biomarkers, ultrasound (subtypes)
Melanoma	Chest x-ray, CT head, MRI ± PET/CT × 3 years (Stages IIb-IV)

REFERENCES

1. DeSantis CE, Lin CC, Mariotto AB, et al. Cancer treatment and survivorship statistics, 2014. *CA Cancer J Clin*. 2014;64(4):252–271.
2. Yourman LC, Lee SJ, Schonberg MA, et al. Prognostic indices for older adults: a systematic review. *JAMA*. 2012;307(2):182–192.
3. Reuben DB, Rosen S, Schickedanz HB. Principles of geriatric assessment. In: Halter JB, Studenski S, High KP, et al., eds. *Hazzard's Geriatric Medicine and Gerontology*. 7th ed. *(Kindle Location 7621)*. New York, NY: McGraw-Hill Education; 2016:157–171.
4. Wildiers H, Heeren P, Puts M, et al. International Society of Geriatric Oncology consensus on geriatric assessment in older patients with cancer. *J Clin Oncol*. 2014;32(24):2595–2603.
5. Mohile SG, Xian Y, Dale W, et al. Association of a cancer diagnosis with vulnerability and frailty in older Medicare beneficiaries. *J Natl Cancer Inst*. 2009;101(17):1206–1215.
6. Bylow K, Mohile SG, Stadler WM, Dale W. Does androgen-deprivation therapy accelerate the development of frailty in older men with prostate cancer?: a conceptual review. *Cancer*. 2007;110(12):2604–2613.
7. Fagard K, Leonard S, Deschodt M, et al. The impact of frailty on postoperative outcomes in individuals aged 65 and over undergoing elective surgery for colorectal cancer: a systematic review. *J Geriatr Oncol*. 2016;7(6):479–491.
8. Ferrucci L, Fabbri L, Walston JD. Frailty. In: Halter JBO, Joseph G, Studenski S, et al, eds. *Hazzard's Geriatric Medicine and Gerontology*. 7th ed. New York, NY: McGraw-Hill Education. Kindle Edition; 2016:Kindle Locations 29246–29248.
9. Society AG. *Geriatrics Review Syllabus: A Core Curriculum in Geriatric Medicine*. New York, NY: American Geriatrics Society; 2016.
10. By the American Geriatrics Society 2015 Beers Criteria Update Expert Panel. American geriatrics society 2015 updated beers criteria for potentially inappropriate medication use in older adults. *J Am Geriatr Soc*. 2015;63(11):2227–2246.
11. Vande Walle N, Kenis C, Heeren P, et al. Fall predictors in older cancer patients: a multicenter prospective study. *BMC Geriatr*. 2014;14:135.
12. Alexander BH, Rivara FP, Wolf ME. The cost and frequency of hospitalization for fall-related injuries in older adults. *Am J Public Health*. 1992;82(7):1020–1023.
13. Lord S. Falls. In: Halter JB, Ouslander JG, Studenski S, et al, eds. *Hazzard's Geriatric Medicine and Gerontology*. New York, NY: McGraw Hill Education; 2016:723–732.
14. Broughman JR, Williams GR, Deal AM, et al. Prevalence of sarcopenia in older patients with colorectal cancer. *J Geriatr Oncol*. 2015;6(6):442–445.
15. Luciani A, Gilda A, Tagliabue L, et al. The impact of chemotherapy on sarcopenia and fatigue in elderly cancer patients: a prospective pilot study. *J Clin Oncol*. 2008;26(suppl 15):9635.
16. Lord S. Falls. In: Halter JB., Ouslander JG, Studenski S, et al., eds. *Hazard's Geriatric Medicine and Gerontology*. 7th ed. New York, NY: McGraw Hill; 2016:724–732.
17. Beaudart C, Zaaria M, Pasleau F, et al. Health outcomes of sarcopenia: a systematic review and meta-analysis. *PLoS ONE [Electronic Resource]*. 2017;12(1):e0169548.
18. Charlton K, Nichols C, Bowden S, et al. Poor nutritional status of older subacute patients predicts clinical outcomes and mortality at 18 months of follow-up. *Eur J Clin Nutr*. 2012;66(11):1224–1228.

19. Shakersain B, Santoni G, Faxen-Irving G, et al. Nutritional status and survival among old adults: an 11-year population-based longitudinal study. *Eur J Clin Nutr.* 2016;70(3):320–325.
20. Neumann SA, Miller MD, Daniels L, et al. Nutritional status and clinical outcomes of older patients in rehabilitation. *J Hum Nutr Diet.* 2005;18(2):129–136.
21. Rasheed S, Woods RT. Malnutrition and quality of life in older people: a systematic review and meta-analysis. *Ageing Res Rev.* 2013;12(2):561–566.
22. Izawa KP, Watanabe S, Oka K, et al. Differences in daily in-hospital physical activity and geriatric nutritional risk index in older cardiac inpatients: preliminary results. *Aging Clin Exp Res.* 2014;26(6):599–605.
23. Murry DJ, Riva L, Poplack DG. Impact of nutrition on pharmacokinetics of anti-neoplastic agents. *Int J Cancer Suppl.* 1998;11:48–51.
24. Versteeg KS, Konings IR, Lagaay AM, et al. Prediction of treatment-related toxicity and outcome with geriatric assessment in elderly patients with solid malignancies treated with chemotherapy: a systematic review. *Ann Oncol.* 2014;25(10):1914–1918.
25. Van Cutsem E, Arends J. The causes and consequences of cancer-associated malnutrition. *Eur J Oncol Nurs.* 2005(9 suppl 2):S51–S63.
26. Arrieta O, Michel Ortega RM, Villanueva-Rodriguez G, et al. Association of nutritional status and serum albumin levels with development of toxicity in patients with advanced non-small cell lung cancer treated with paclitaxel-cisplatin chemotherapy: a prospective study. *BMC Cancer.* 2010;10:50.
27. Chandra RK. Nutrition and the immune system: an introduction. *Am J Clin Nutr.* 1997;66(2):460S–463S.
28. Braunschweig C, Gomez S, Sheean PM. Impact of declines in nutritional status on outcomes in adult patients hospitalized for more than 7 days. *J Am Diet Assoc.* 2000;100(11):1316–1322; quiz 1323–1314.
29. Gout BS, Barker LA, Crowe TC. Malnutrition identification, diagnosis and dietetic referrals: Are we doing a good enough job? *Nutr Diet.* 2009;66(4):206–211.
30. Neumayer LA, Smout RJ, Horn HG, et al. Early and sufficient feeding reduces length of stay and charges in surgical patients. *J Surg Res.* 2001;95(1):73–77.
31. Argiles JM. Cancer-associated malnutrition. *Eur J Oncol Nurs.* 2005(9 suppl 2):S39–S50.
32. Laviano A, Meguid MM. Nutritional issues in cancer management. *Nutrition.* 1996;12(5):358–371.
33. Attar A, Malka D, Sabate JM, et al. Malnutrition is high and underestimated during chemotherapy in gastrointestinal cancer: an AGEO prospective cross-sectional multicenter study. *Nutr Cancer.* 2012;64(4):535–542.
34. Wells JL, Dumbrell AC. Nutrition and aging: assessment and treatment of compromised nutritional status in frail elderly patients. *Clin Interv Aging.* 2006;1(1):67–79.
35. Wrisley DM, Kauffman TL. Balance testing and training. In: *A Comprehensive Guide to Geriatric Rehabilitation.* 3rd ed. London: Churchill Livingston; 2014:433–438.
36. Kenny R, Rubenstein L, Tinetti M, et al. Summary of the updated American Geriatrics Society/British Geriatrics Society clinical practice guideline for prevention of falls in older persons. *J Am Geriatr Soc.* 2011;59:148–157.
37. Lee SH, Kim HS. Exercise intervention for preventing falls among older people in care facilities: a meta-analysis. *Worldviews Evid Based Nurs.* 2017;14(1):74–80.
38. Stubbs B, Brefka S, Denkinger MD. What works to prevent falls in community-dwelling older adults? Umbrella review of meta-analyses of randomized controlled trials. *Phys Ther.* 2015;95:1095–1110.

39. Sherrington C, Whitney JC, Lord SR, et al. Effective exercise for the prevention of falls: a systematic review and meta-analysis. *J Am Geriatr Soc*. 2008;56:2234–2243.
40. World Health Organization. *Global Health Report on Falls Prevention*. Geneva, Switzerland, 2007.
41. Park J, Hughes AK. Nonpharmacological approaches to the management of chronic pain in community-dwelling older adults: a review of empirical evidence. *J Am Geriatr Soc*. 2012;60(3):555–568. doi: 10.1111/j.1532-5415.2011.03846.x

7 Late-Term Effects of Cancer Therapy on Older Adult Cancer Survivors

Beatrice J. Edwards
Linda Pang
Maria Suarez Almazor

Late effects of cancer and its treatments in adults 65 years of age and older often exacerbate disabilities and chronic conditions associated with the aging process. Cancer treatment affects various body systems, which contributes to the complexity of providing care to older cancer survivors. Effects on the central and peripheral nervous systems, for example, include cognitive impairment, peripheral neuropathy, and balance or gait disorders. Cancer therapy also can cause cardiotoxicity, resulting in cardiomyopathies and accelerated ischemic disease. Sensory organ ototoxicity, a common side effect of cisplatin treatment that can lead to permanent hearing loss, is another condition related to cancer treatment. The endocrine system also is affected by cancer therapies that can lead to late effects such as metabolic syndrome, diabetes, hyperlipidemia, and ischemic heart disease. The musculoskeletal system is also affected by cancer therapies; patients become more susceptible to accelerated bone loss, low bone mass, osteoporosis, and fractures.

On a psychological level, a cancer diagnosis and associated treatment can increase a survivor's risk for depression and anxiety. Cancer and its treatment can also result in erectile dysfunction, hypogonadism, and dyspareunia. In addition to all of these late effects, cancer survivors are at higher risk for recurrent or secondary malignancies. This chapter discusses the most common late-term effects resulting from cancer and/or its treatment that must be addressed while assessing older adults and managing their care. In this chapter, *older adults* will refer to those ages 65 and older.

CARDIOTOXICITY

Although there are limited data on cardiotoxicity specific to adults ages 65 and older, this is an area of interest (1–3). The combination of the aging process and cardiac dysfunction associated with treatment increases the need to carefully monitor patients who received high-dose anthracycline or radiotherapy treatment. Preexisting cardiac conditions such as valvular disease, history of myocardial infarction, or other cardiovascular risk factors predispose patients with cancer to more severe adverse cardiac events. Cardiotoxicity may manifest as new or worsening hypertension, cardiac ischemia, or heart failure. Bevacizumab is associated with new or worsening hypertension. Anthracyclines, paclitaxel, or trastuzumab can cause cardiotoxicity, left ventricular function dysfunction, or heart failure. Radiation, paclitaxel, antimetabolites, and targeted agents such as bevacizumab contribute to ischemic heart disease. Arrhythmias may be caused by arsenic trioxide and most antiemetics. Older adults are at particularly high risk for cardiotoxicity because risk for age-related heart failure increases with age. Androgen-deprivation therapy (ADT) may make men more susceptible to cardiotoxicity (3). The risk of dying from cardiac causes increases each year for patients receiving ADT. One study revealed that cardiac-related prostate cancer mortality was 5% among men receiving ADT versus 2% in those who only had surgery (3). Cardiotoxicity also may be directly responsible for adverse clinical outcomes (2,3).

BONE LOSS AND OSTEOPOROSIS

Cancer survivors ages 65 and older are at higher risk for osteoporosis, falls, and fall-related injuries than the general population. Factors contributing to this risk include increased age, decreased muscle mass and strength, and bone mineral density (BMD). Fall-related fractures in older adults are associated with hip fractures, disability, morbidity, and increased mortality. The negative consequences of hip fractures such as decreased mobility and interference with daily living activities or self-care substantially interfere with recovery of function and quality of life. Fall screening and prevention is needed because mortality is heightened among older women and men after hip fracture. Evidence indicates that adults older than age 65 are at a 5- to 8-fold increased risk for dying during the first 3 months after a fracture (4). Research also suggests that 20% to 30% of patients with hip fractures die during the first 12 months after sustaining the fracture (5).

Breast cancer is associated with chemotherapy-induced menopause in perimenopausal women and accelerated bone loss. Upon diagnosis, women with breast cancer who were enrolled in the Women's Health Initiative were at a 50% increased risk for hip fracture (6). Chemotherapy use also results in increased risk for fractures among women with breast cancer (7). In addition, adjuvant hormone therapy such as aromatase inhibitors will result in bone loss and subsequent fractures (8). Men with prostate cancer who receive ADT will also experience accelerated bone loss and are at increased risk for osteoporosis attributable to advanced age, poor nutrition, and vitamin D deficiency (9). A group of Danish investigators who conducted a nationwide register study found that prostate cancer was associated with increased risk for fractures (1.8-fold for all fractures and 3.7-fold for hip fractures) (9). These investigators found that higher hip fracture risk became apparent soon after diagnosis and remained pronounced even among long-term survivors. Their results further suggested that ADT and orchiectomy were associated with a 1.7-fold higher risk for fractures in addition to the overall fracture risk (9).

Mortality after fractures among men who have had prostate cancer is substantially increased, as seen in a Surveillance, Epidemiology, and End Results-Medicare study in which men with fractures who received ADT had an adjusted death risk that was twice as high as for men who did not receive ADT (10). National Comprehensive Cancer Network Guidelines recommend BMD testing in women or men who will receive adjuvant hormonal therapy (11). Considering that older adults have a higher prevalence of low bone mass and osteoporosis, National Osteoporosis Foundation clinical guidelines should be followed, and men and women 65 years and older with cancer should undergo bone densitometry and appropriate treatment (12).

Two clinical trials support the recommendation that patients with breast or prostate cancer and low bone mass (osteopenia) or osteoporosis receive antiresorptive therapy. A trial conducted by Smith et al. found that men with prostate cancer who were receiving ADT had a T-score of −1.0 or lower (13). A multicenter randomized study also reported that treatment with denosumab reduced risk for vertebral fractures by 62% for women with breast cancer and normal or low bone mass (osteopenia) who were starting aromatase inhibitors and reduced overall fracture risk by 50% (14).

MD Anderson recommends BMD testing for all older adults who have a life expectancy longer than 5 years. Patients should consume a calcium-rich diet and take calcium supplements (e.g., calcium citrate with vitamin D 600 mg daily) in addition to vitamin D3 1,000 to 2,000 units/d. Total calcium intake including diet and supplements should be 1,200 mg/d. Older adults who have low bone mass or osteoporosis will benefit from antiresorptive therapy in the form of bisphosphonates or denosumab to reduce fracture risk. Among the antiresorptive medications, denosumab has been shown to reduce risk for vertebral and other fractures (14). For survivors undergoing active cancer care (chemotherapy and/or adjuvant hormonal or possible immunotherapy), BMD should be repeated on a yearly basis; for survivors no longer under active care, BMD testing should be ordered every 2 years (15). Use of anabolic agents such as teriparatide is not recommended for cancer survivors with a history of radiation therapy.

COGNITIVE IMPAIRMENT

Cognitive impairment and dementia may be seen in older adult cancer survivors. The effects of chemotherapy on cognitive processes likely will be superimposed on age-related mild cognitive impairment. The prevalence of dementia increases with age, from 5% among those ages 71 to 79 to 37.4% among those age 90 and older (16). However, primary care clinicians may not recognize cognitive impairment during routine history and physical examinations. As a result, most patients do not receive an accurate diagnosis until they are in the moderate to severe stages of disease. Chemotherapy-related cognitive impairment is another concern. Most often, poor attention, recall, and difficulty performing instrumental activities of daily living (ADLs) are cited. Aromatase inhibitors and ADT can further affect cognitive function. Domains affected include verbal, verbal memory, verbal functioning, and informational processing speed. In some cases, cognitive impairment may improve upon completion of therapy.

Mild cognitive impairment or dementia treatment usually necessitates efforts of a team that includes geriatricians, social workers, and physical and occupational therapists. Cognitive enhancers are now recommended for patients who need cranial radiation. Home safety is of paramount importance; as dementia progresses, patients will require increasingly supervised living arrangements.

ARTHRITIS

Musculoskeletal disorders are widely prevalent in the general population. The prevalence of these disorders increases with age, and they are among major comorbid conditions affecting quality of life among elderly people (17). Preexisting rheumatic conditions such as osteoarthritis or rheumatoid arthritis cause pain and functional impairments that can substantially contribute to the comorbidity burden of cancer survivors (18).

AROMATASE INHIBITOR–INDUCED ARTHRALGIA AND MUSCULOSKELETAL PAIN

Aromatase inhibitors are an essential therapy for women with estrogen-positive breast cancer. A major adverse event associated with these agents is arthralgia, which can occur in as many as 40% of patients and can be severe and limiting, resulting in poor adherence and drug discontinuation (19). Patients may experience pain in large and small joints and/or tendinitis, most commonly in the hands, which can cause trigger finger or de Quervain's tenosynovitis. These symptoms are particularly challenging for patients with preexisting joint conditions such as osteoarthritis. Nonsteroidal anti-inflammatory drugs (NSAIDs) are the treatment mainstay, but, for elderly patients, practitioners must exercise caution and consider preexisting renal and/or cardiovascular diseases when prescribing these agents. For patients with severe symptoms, switching therapy to tamoxifen may be appropriate. Patients receiving aromatase inhibitors also are at increased risk for bone loss, osteoporosis, and fractures.

RADIATION-INDUCED FIBROSIS

Many patients develop progressive local soft-tissue fibrosis after radiation therapy that can result in substantial disability and limited mobility, which is of particular concern for elderly cancer survivors (20). Damage to neuromuscular tissues (muscle, plexus, and nerves) results in progressive limitations that vary according to the location, structures involved, and degree of fibrosis. It is challenging to manage these syndromes. Fibrosis also can cause pain in adjacent structures because of impaired mobility. Physical therapy can somewhat limit range of motion loss progression, but it is difficult to recuperate any existing deficits. Rehabilitation and occupational therapy can assist with adaptation strategies to improve ADLs (21).

FIBROMYALGIA

Cancer survivors, especially women, are at higher risk for fibromyalgia (22,23). Symptoms include widespread pain, poor sleep, fatigue, and tenderness over multiple tendinous insertions. Fibromyalgia is a poorly understood syndrome. Patients experience decreased tolerance to pain that is thought to be primarily central. Few treatments improve this condition, so nonpharmacological management is important (24). Patients should be encouraged to engage in regular exercise, which has proven beneficial in various clinical trials and is the only therapeutic approach associated with strong evidence for efficacy, according to guidelines. Drug therapies have weak efficacy. Acetaminophen, NSAIDs, and opioids generally are not very effective. Therapeutic options include serotonin norepinephrine reuptake inhibitors, selective serotonin reuptake inhibitors, tricyclic antidepressants (considering that nortriptyline is preferred for elderly people), and pregabalin. Fibromyalgia is a chronic condition, and its treatment necessitates patient education and lifestyle changes regarding sleep and exercise habits. This is especially important for older cancer survivors for whom use of psychotropic drugs may result in deleterious outcomes, and these drugs may interact with other pharmacological therapies.

MYOSITIS

Polymyositis and dermatomyositis can develop as a paraneoplastic syndrome with many tumors (25). Clinical manifestations include profound proximal muscle weakness, which in severe cases can result in dysphagia, hoarseness, and shortness of breath. Patients with dermatomyositis also develop a distinctive rash. Paraneoplastic myositis generally is associated with advanced metastatic disease, and its course is dependent upon tumor progression. Most patients are treated with glucocorticoids, and occasionally, for those who do not respond, intravenous immunoglobulin. In general, prognosis is poor because of the advanced cancer stage associated with this syndrome. However, for survivors for whom cancer therapy is successful, the inflammatory components of myositis likely will resolve. Nevertheless, many patients, especially those who are elderly, may experience muscle weakness because of muscular fibrosis and atrophy that can be aggravated by chronic steroid therapy that can cause myopathy. For these patients, drug therapy is not required because they present with "burnt-out" disease; rehabilitation and physical therapy are the major treatment components (25).

IMMUNOTHERAPY-RELATED ADVERSE EVENTS

Immunotherapy has revolutionized cancer treatment. Immune checkpoint inhibitors are increasingly used to treat various cancers to increase antitumoral immunity with impressive efficacy. However, because of immune function enhancement, many patients develop immunity-related adverse events that can be severe and result in death. These include rash, colitis, endocrinopathies, pneumonitis, arthritis, and myositis, among many others (26). Although many of these adverse events resolve with discontinuation of the checkpoint inhibitor and immunosuppressive therapy, such as glucocorticoids, some effects and sequelae can persist. There are several reports of severe arthritis that persists after therapy discontinuation. Because these agents are being used for longer periods of time, and possibly for maintenance therapy, these events may occur more frequently in cancer survivors. The primary therapy for patients with arthritis has been glucocorticoids, but clinicians should be mindful of the deleterious effects of chronic steroid therapy, especially in older patients, such as bone loss, diabetes, and hypertension. Because this is an evolving field, more clinical experience is needed to develop recommendations on ways to best manage these therapy complications in elderly patients.

BALANCE AND GAIT DISORDERS

Cancer survivors ages 65 and older are at elevated risk for falls and disorders in their gait and balance because almost all body systems are affected by complications associated with cancer and its treatment (27). Multiple factors contribute to impaired balance and gait including underlying medical conditions; interactions associated with use of multiple medications; and impairments in sensory, motor, and central processing systems. It is important to integrate screening and surveillance assessments into clinical practice and to discuss fall prevention interventions to address these functional threats during patient–provider encounters. Balance may also be affected by chemotherapy-induced peripheral neuropathy (CIPN) (28–30), which may contribute to balance disorders and falls because sensory input from lower extremities is greatly affected.

SARCOPENIA

An age-associated loss of muscle mass and strength—sarcopenia—begins at around the fifth decade of life (31). Sarcopenia, which can contribute to negative health outcomes including an increased risk for falls and fractures and metabolic diseases such as type 2 diabetes mellitus, may increase the necessity for assisted living placement. Linear sarcopenic declines in muscle mass and strength are, however, punctuated by transient periods of muscle disuse that can accelerate loss of muscle and strength, which can result in increased risk for sarcopenia. Muscle disuse may be expected with bed rest or immobilization (e.g., disuse attributable to surgery or acute illness requiring hospitalization); however, research has shown that even a relative reduction in ambulation (reduced daily steps) results in significant reductions in muscle mass and strength and possibly an increase in disease risk (32). Investigators have documented that 2 to 3 weeks of reduced daily steps may induce negative changes in body composition, a reduction in muscle strength and quality, anabolic resistance, and decrements in glycemic control in older adults (31,32). Of importance, periods of reduced ambulation are common and can increase full recovery difficulty, especially for older adults (32). Muscle loss is associated with denervation on electrophysiologic studies and type 2 atrophy on muscle biopsy. In addition to loss of strength and muscle bulk, changes in speed and coordination of movement increase with advancing age. Chemotherapy results in a decline in muscle mass not explained by a decline in body mass index (BMI). Patients with sarcopenia likely will experience substantial muscle loss during cancer care. For survivors, management likely will involve exercise, a high-protein diet, and (ideally) strength training.

PSYCHOLOGIC EFFECTS

The effect of cancer on the psychologic sphere is considerable, so cancer survivors may experience depression and anxiety many years after their cancer diagnosis. Most women with gynecologic cancers express a need for emotional support, but only 37% of them receive such support. Major depression also is seen in cancer survivors and often is accompanied by anxiety. Chapter 4 provides details about assessing and managing cancer survivors' emotional health.

METABOLIC SYNDROME

Certain cancer therapies such as hormone-modifying, androgen-suppressing, or anti-estrogen treatments place cancer survivors at elevated risk for posttreatment metabolic syndrome (33). The consequences of metabolic syndrome includes cardiovascular disease, nonalcoholic steatohepatitis, diabetes, and sleep disturbance. It is important for primary care providers to closely monitor the lipid profiles, liver enzymes, and markers of glycemic function in patients who have been treated with antiestrogen therapy or androgen suppression therapy (this particularly is applicable for men and women with hypogonadism). Men with prostate cancer who received ADT are at increased risk for insulin resistance and dyslipidemia—both are indicators of metabolic syndrome. ADT for 12 months results in a decrease in lean muscle mass and an increase in body weight, fat mass, and waist circumference. In a similar fashion, women with breast cancer who receive chemotherapy are at elevated risk for weight gain, increased body fat, and a decline in lean muscle mass. Breast cancer survivors with metabolic syndrome are at higher risk for cancer recurrence than those without metabolic syndrome.

FATIGUE

Fatigue, one of the most common side effects associated with cancer therapy, can negatively influence quality of life. Cancer therapy-related fatigue does not improve with rest or sleep. Fatigue often is caused by therapy modalities, anemia, nutritional deficiencies, depression, sleep disorders, and medications. Some medications such as anxiolytics, tranquilizers, and narcotics can contribute to fatigue. American Society of Clinical Oncology guidelines recommend that all patients should be screened for fatigue from the point of diagnosis onward (34). Healthcare providers should assess fatigue history, disease status, and treatable contributing factors. All patients should be educated about differences between normal and cancer-related fatigue, causes of fatigue, and contributing factors. Patients should be educated about strategies to manage fatigue including physical activity, psychosocial interventions such as cognitive and behavioral therapies and psychoeducational therapies, and mind–body interventions such as yoga and acupuncture (34).

CHEMOTHERAPY-INDUCED PERIPHERAL NEUROPATHY

Chemotherapy and its side effects such as weakness, CIPN, and problems with balance and walking ability increase cancer survivors' risk for falls (28–30). Men with prostate cancer who receive ADT and who are older than age 70 are at especially high risk. Taxanes and platinum agents most commonly cause neuropathy; vinca alkaloids also can cause CIPN. Patients with preexisting neuropathy are at elevated risk for CIPN (29). Because of the lack of high-quality evidence, no established agents are recommended to prevent CIPN in people with cancer who are undergoing treatment with neurotoxic agents. These agents should not be offered to prevent CIPN: acetyl-L-carnitine, amifostine, amitriptyline, calcium acetate/magnesium carbonate, diethyldithiocarbamate, glutathione, nimodipine, Org 2766, all-trans retinoic acid, recombinant human leukemia inhibitory factor, and vitamin E. CIPN clinicians may offer duloxetine, however. Although there is no strong evidence of benefit associated with use of tricyclic antidepressants; gabapentin; and a topical gel containing baclofen, amitriptyline, and ketamine, it may be reasonable to try these agents in select patients (29). Considering the increased risk for falls in this populations and the high likelihood of comorbid conditions and mixed diagnoses, clinicians should assess survivors' fall risk.

OTOTOXICITY

Hearing loss attributable to noise exposure, injury, or age-related changes is a common condition in older adults. For cancer survivors who have been treated with antineoplastic treatments such as platinum agents, chemotherapy, and radiation or surgery that involves the ear or auditory nerves, ototoxicity exacerbates this problem (35). The combined effects of these conditions can have a substantial impact on the social and physical lives of older adults who often are at risk for isolation and falls. Standardized guidelines outline best practices for long-term follow-up of this condition among cancer survivors. The guidelines are stratified according to age and the type of therapy used to treat the cancer. For patients with head and neck cancer who are treated with radiotherapy, for example, ongoing monitoring every 5 years is advised unless more frequent monitoring is clinically indicated. Baseline auditory assessment is recommended for all cancer survivors who receive any platinum chemotherapy (35).

EXERCISES DECREASE RISK FOR NEW OR RECURRENT CANCERS

A growing body of research shows that physical activity and structured exercise interventions can enhance the physical and psychological function of cancer survivors (36–39). Despite the evidence, physicians and other healthcare providers often miss the opportunity to discuss the benefits of exercise with survivors (40).

One study of colon and lung cancer survivors found that certain subgroups including those 65 years of age and older were more likely to not have had exercise-related discussions with their physicians. Several studies focusing on cancer survivors 65 years of age and older support the positive effects of exercise and recommend tailoring exercise interventions to cancer diagnosis, cognitive status, comorbid conditions, and level of physical mobility or function (37,38,41).

Breast cancer. Although risk reduction varies (20%–80%), most studies suggest that 30 to 60 minutes of moderate- to high-intensity exercise per day lowers breast cancer risk. Among women with breast cancer, physical activity can improve function, muscle strength and mass, and body size. Exercise also helps alter endogenous estrogen, insulin, and C-reactive protein levels—all factors associated with better survival (38).

Colon cancer. Physical activity can lower a person's risk for colon cancer (42). Recommendations can involve mobile eHealth interventions, strength training, or other forms of activity that decrease the amount of time of being inactive or sedentary. A decrease in colon cancer risk can be achieved regardless of BMI, and people who are most active benefit the most.

Endometrial, lung, and ovarian cancers. Women who are physically active have a 20% to 40% reduced risk for endometrial cancer versus those who do not exercise. Higher levels of physical activity also protect against lung cancer (as high as a 20% risk reduction), particularly among men. Physical activity also may reduce ovarian and prostate cancer risks (43).

OLDER ADULTS AND PAIN

Persistent pain, especially in cognitively impaired older adults, often goes undertreated (Table 7.1) (44–46). When assessing older adults for pain, bear in mind that they may be reluctant or unable to report their pain; consequently, clinicians must maintain diligence when assessing pain perception during office visits. They should use simple pain tools or ask questions that solicit yes/no answers to prompt self-reports of pain in people with moderate cognitive impairment. Patients with severe cognitive impairment cannot verbally express pain but can be evaluated for pain-related behaviors. Common pain behaviors seen in cognitively impaired older adults include changes in facial expression such as a slight frown, grimacing, a winkled forehead, closed or tightened eyes, changes in verbalizations or vocalizations (such as sighing, moaning, or verbal abuse), changes in body movements (fidgeting or rigid or tense body posture), or changes in activity patterns or routines such as appetite changes.

Pain assessment should include a psychosocial assessment and an evaluation for depression and anxiety, both of which can coexist or worsen pain symptoms. A pain assessment also can focus on educating family members to observe the patient for extreme drowsiness, overuse or abuse of pain medications, or reluctance to use medication because of fear of addiction. A functional assessment also should be performed to evaluate the ways in which pain affects a patient's ability to perform ADLs, general activity level, and quality of life.

TABLE 7.1 Nondrug Intervention to Address Persistent Pain in Older Adults

Intervention	Outcomes	Problems Studied
Physical		
Exercise (walking, tai chi, and yoga)	Positive	Lower extremity osteoarthritis, chronic low back pain, chronic pain
Acupuncture	Positive	Back, knee, shoulder, neck
Transcutaneous electrical nerve stimulation	Uncertain	Knee, back
Qigong	Uncertain	Back, neck
Massage	Positive	Back, neck
Psychosocial		
Cognitive behavioral training	Positive	Chronic pain
Guided imagery with progressive muscle relaxation	Positive	Chronic osteoarthritis pain
Music	Positive	Chronic pain
Mindfulness-based meditation	Uncertain	Chronic low back pain
Self-management education	Positive	Chronic pain, chronic low back pain

Sources: From Boland EG, Ahmedzai SH. Persistent pain in cancer survivors. *Curr Opin Support Palliat Care.* 2017;11(3):181–190; Makris UE, Abrams RC, Gurland B, et al. Management of persistent pain in the older patient: a clinical review. *JAMA.* 2014;312(8):825–836; Park J, Hughes AK. Nonpharmacological approaches to the management of chronic pain in community-dwelling older adults: a review of empirical evidence. *J Am Geriatr Soc.* 2012;60(3):555–568.

Providers must work with patients and their family members to create goals for optimal balance in pain relief, functional improvement, and adverse events. For older adults, consider nondrug options early in their treatment plan. Use local treatments to address local pain (e.g., manipulation, massage, heat, physical therapy, and transcutaneous electrical nerve stimulation), topical anesthetics, or steroid joint injections. Encourage healthy behaviors such as regular physical activity, which can decrease pain scores, improve mood, and boost functional status. A referral to a pain clinic for an interdisciplinary team approach may be useful for patients who have complex pain syndromes or a poor response to first-line treatments. Interdisciplinary team members may also incorporate cognitive techniques into the treatment plan such as biofeedback, music and pet therapy, and systematic desensitization.

When beginning a pain management regimen for adults ages 65 and older, it is important to select medications with the lowest adverse effect profile. For mild pain, consider scheduled doses of acetaminophen. NSAIDs can be more effective for inflammatory pain but are associated with more adverse events including renal dysfunction, gastrointestinal bleeding, fluid retention, and heart failure, which can limit the treatment of persistent pain in older adults with comorbidities. Topical NSAIDs appear to be safe and effective in the short term. Providers also can consider topical analgesics such as a lidocaine patch or a counter-stimulant such as a capsaicin patch. For moderate to severe pain, providers may need to consider opioid treatments; however, do not prescribe opioid analgesics as long-term treatment for chronic noncancer pain unless risks are discussed with the patient. Opioid-related risks include falls or fractures, hospitalization relative NSAID use, and constipation. Initiate opioids at low doses and up-titrate with caution.

REFERENCES

1. Reddy P, Shenoy C, Blaes AH. Cardio-oncology in the older adult. *J Geriatr Oncol.* 2017;8(4):308–314. doi:10.1016/j.jgo.2017.04.001
2. Pinder MC, Duan Z, Goodwin JS, et al. Congestive heart failure in older women treated with adjuvant anthracycline chemotherapy for breast cancer. *J Clin Oncol.* 2007;25(25):3808–3815. doi:10.1200/JCO.2006.10.4976
3. Tsai HK, D'Amico AV, Sadetsky N, et al. Androgen deprivation therapy for localized prostate cancer and the risk of cardiovascular mortality. *J Natl Cancer Inst.* 2007;99(20):1516–1524. doi:10.1093/jnci/djm168
4. Haentjens P, Magaziner J, Colon-Emeric CS, et al. Meta-analysis: excess mortality after hip fracture among older women and men. *Ann Intern Med.* 2010;152(6):380–390. doi:10.7326/0003-4819-152-6-201003160-00008
5. Cenzer IS, Tang V, Boscardin WJ, et al. One-year mortality after hip fracture: development and validation of a prognostic index. *J Am Geriatr Soc.* 2016;64(9):1863–1868. doi:10.1111/jgs.14237
6. Chen Z, Maricic M, Aragaki AK, et al. Fracture risk increases after diagnosis of breast or other cancers in postmenopausal women: results from the Women's Health Initiative. *Osteoporos Int.* 2009;20(4):527–536. doi:10.1007/s00198-008-0721-0
7. Edwards BJ, Gradishar WJ, Smith ME, et al. Elevated incidence of fractures in women with invasive breast cancer. *Osteoporos Int.* 2016;27(2):499–507. doi:10.1007/s00198-015-3246-3
8. Eastell R, Adams J, Clack G, et al. Long-term effects of anastrozole on bone mineral density: 7-year results from the ATAC trial. *Ann Oncol.* 2011;22(4):857–862. doi:10.1093/annonc/mdq541
9. Abrahamsen B, Nielsen MF, Eskildsen P, et al. Fracture risk in Danish men with prostate cancer: a nationwide register study. *BJU Int.* 2007;100(4):749–754. doi:10.1111/j.1464-410X.2007.07163.x
10. Beebe-Dimmer JL, Cetin K, Shahinian V, et al. Timing of androgen deprivation therapy use and fracture risk among elderly men with prostate cancer in the United States. *Pharmacoepidemiol Drug Saf.* 2012;21(1):70–78. doi:10.1002/pds.2258
11. Gralow JR, Biermann JS, Farooki A, et al. NCCN Task Force Report: bone health in cancer care. *J Natl Compr Canc Netw.* 2013;11(suppl 3):S1–S50; quiz S51. doi:10.6004/JNCCN.2013.0215
12. Cosman F, de Beur SJ, LeBoff MS, et al. Clinician's guide to prevention and treatment of osteoporosis. *Osteoporos Int.* 2014;25(10):2359–2381. doi:10.1007/s00198-014-2794-2
13. Smith MR, Egerdie B, Hernandez Toriz N, et al. Denosumab in men receiving androgen-deprivation therapy for prostate cancer. *N Engl J Med.* 2009;361(8):745–755. doi:10.1056/NEJMoa0809003

14. Gnant M, Pfeiler G, Dubsky PC, et al. Adjuvant denosumab in breast cancer (ABCSG-18): a multicentre, randomised, double-blind, placebo-controlled trial. *Lancet.* 2015;386(9992):433–443. doi:10.1016/S0140-6736(15)60995-3

15. National Osteoporosis Foundation. Clinician's guide to prevention and treatment of osteoporosis. Available at: https://cdn.nof.org/wp-content/uploads/2016/01/995.pdf. doi:10.1007/s00198-014-2794-2

16. Laurin D, Masaki KH, Foley DJ, et al. Midlife dietary intake of antioxidants and risk of late-life incident dementia: the Honolulu-Asia Aging Study. *Am J Epidemiol.* 2004;159(10):959–967. doi:10.1093/aje/kwh124

17. Michet CJ Jr, Evans JM, Fleming KC, et al. Common rheumatologic diseases in elderly patients. *Mayo Clin Proc.* 1995;70(12):1205–1214. doi:10.1016/S0025-6196(11)63449-6

18. Kenzik KM, Kent EE, Martin MY, et al. Chronic condition clusters and functional impairment in older cancer survivors: a population-based study. *J Cancer Surviv.* 2016;10(6):1096–1103. doi:10.1007/s11764-016-0553-4

19. Coleman RE, Bolten WW, Lansdown M, et al. Aromatase inhibitor-induced arthralgia: clinical experience and treatment recommendations. *Cancer Treat Rev.* 2008;34(3):275–282. doi:10.1016/j.ctrv.2007.10.004

20. Stubblefield MD. Radiation fibrosis syndrome: neuromuscular and musculoskeletal complications in cancer survivors. *PM R.* 2011;3(11):1041–1054. doi:10.1016/j.pmrj.2011.08.535

21. Stubblefield MD. Clinical evaluation and management of radiation fibrosis syndrome. *Phys Med Rehabil Clin N Am.* 2017;28(1):89–100. doi:10.1016/j.pmr.2016.08.003

22. Schou Bredal I, Smeby NA, Ottesen S, et al. Chronic pain in breast cancer survivors: comparison of psychosocial, surgical, and medical characteristics between survivors with and without pain. *J Pain Symptom Manage.* 2014;48(5):852–862. doi:10.1016/j.jpainsymman.2013.12.239

23. Akkaya N, Atalay NS, Selcuk ST, et al. Frequency of fibromyalgia syndrome in breast cancer patients. *Int J Clin Oncol.* 2013;18(2):285–292. doi:10.1007/s10147-012-0377-9

24. Macfarlane GJ, Kronisch C, Dean LE, et al. EULAR revised recommendations for the management of fibromyalgia. *Ann Rheum Dis.* 2017;76(2):318–328. doi:10.1136/annrheumdis-2016-209724

25. Tiniakou E, Mammen AL. Idiopathic inflammatory myopathies and malignancy: a comprehensive review. *Clin Rev Allergy Immunol.* 2017;52(1):20–33. doi:10.1007/s12016-015-8511-x

26. Suarez-Almazor ME, Kim ST, Abdel-Wahab N, et al. Immune-related adverse events with use of checkpoint inhibitors for immunotherapy of cancer. *Arthritis Rheumatol.* 2017;69(4):687–699. doi:10.1002/art.40043

27. Huang MH, Lytle T, Miller KA, et al. History of falls, balance performance, and quality of life in older cancer survivors. *Gait Posture.* 2014;40(3):451–456. doi:10.1016/j.gaitpost.2014.05.015

28. Miaskowski C, Mastick J, Paul SM, et al. Impact of chemotherapy-induced neurotoxicities on adult cancer survivors' symptom burden and quality of life. *J Cancer Surviv.* 2017. doi:10.1007/s11764-017-0662-8

29. Hershman DL, Lacchetti C, Dworkin RH, et al. Prevention and management of chemotherapy-induced peripheral neuropathy in survivors of adult cancers: American Society of Clinical Oncology Clinical Practice Guideline. *J Clin Oncol.* 2014;32(18):1941–1967. doi:10.1200/JCO.2013.54.0914

30. Cavaletti G, Marmiroli P. Chemotherapy-induced peripheral neurotoxicity. *Curr Opin Neurol*. 2015;28(5):500–507. doi:10.1097/WCO.0000000000000234

31. Zargar H, Almassi N, Kovac E, et al. Change in psoas muscle volume as a predictor of outcomes in patients treated with chemotherapy and radical cystectomy for muscle-invasive bladder cancer. *Bladder Cancer*. 2017;3(1):57–63. doi:10.3233/BLC-160080

32. Bell KE, von Allmen MT, Devries MC, et al. Muscle disuse as a pivotal problem in sarcopenia-related muscle loss and dysfunction. *J Frailty Aging*. 2016;5(1):33–41. doi:10.14283/jfa.2016.78

33. Redig AJ, Munshi HG. Metabolic syndrome after hormone-modifying therapy: risks associated with antineoplastic therapy. *Oncology (Williston Park)*. 2010;24(9):839–844. doi:10.1016/j.amjmed.2009.06.022

34. Bower JE, Bak K, Berger A, et al. Screening, assessment, and management of fatigue in adult survivors of cancer: an American Society of Clinical Oncology Clinical Practice Guideline adaptation. *J Clin Oncol*. 2014;32(17):1840–1850. doi:10.1200/JCO.2013.53.4495

35. Landier W. Ototoxicity and cancer therapy. *Cancer*. 2016;122(11):1647–1658. doi:10.1002/cncr.29779

36. Kilari D, Soto-Perez-de-Celis E, Mohile SG, et al. Designing exercise clinical trials for older adults with cancer: recommendations from 2015 Cancer and Aging Research Group NCI U13 Meeting. *J Geriatr Oncol*. 2016;7(4):293–304. doi:10.1016/j.jgo.2016.04.007

37. Daum CW, Cochrane SK, Fitzgerald JD, et al. Exercise interventions for preserving physical function among cancer survivors in middle to late life. *J Frailty Aging*. 2016;5(4):214–224. doi:10.14283/jfa.2016.92

38. Maliniak ML, Patel AV, McCullough ML, et al. Obesity, physical activity, and breast cancer survival among older breast cancer survivors in the Cancer Prevention Study-II Nutrition Cohort. *Breast Cancer Res Treat*. 2017. doi:10.1007/s10549-017-4470-7

39. Schmitz KH, Courneya KS, Matthews C, et al. American College of Sports Medicine roundtable on exercise guidelines for cancer survivors. *Med Sci Sports Exerc*. 2010;42(7):1409–1426. doi:10.1249/MSS.0b013e3181e0c112

40. Kenzik K, Pisu M, Fouad MN, et al. Are long-term cancer survivors and physicians discussing health promotion and healthy behaviors? *J Cancer Surviv*. 2016;10(2):271–279. doi:10.1007/s11764-015-0473-8

41. Klepin HD, Mohile SG, Mihalko S. Exercise for older cancer patients: feasible and helpful? *Interdiscip Top Gerontol*. 2013;38:146–157. doi:10.1159/000343597

42. Mayer DK, Landucci G, Awoyinka L, et al. SurvivorCHESS to increase physical activity in colon cancer survivors: can we get them moving? *J Cancer Surviv*. 2017. doi:10.1007/s11764-017-0647-7

43. Demark-Wahnefried W, Schmitz KH, Alfano CM, et al. Weight management and physical activity throughout the cancer care continuum. *CA Cancer J Clin*. 2017. doi:10.3322/caac.21441

44. Park J, Hughes AK. Nonpharmacological approaches to the management of chronic pain in community-dwelling older adults: a review of empirical evidence. *J Am Geriatr Soc*. 2012;60(3):555–568. doi:10.1111/j.1532-5415.2011.03846.x

45. Makris UE, Abrams RC, Gurland B, et al. Management of persistent pain in the older patient: a clinical review. *JAMA*. 2014;312(8):825–836. doi:10.1001/jama.2014.9405

46. Boland EG, Ahmedzai SH. Persistent pain in cancer survivors. *Curr Opin Support Palliat Care*. 2017;11(3):181–190. doi:10.1097/SPC.0000000000000292

Management of Site-Specific Cancers

8 Integrative Medicine in Survivorship Care

Gabriel Lopez
Wenli Liu
Alejandro Chaoul
M. Kay Garcia
Lorenzo Cohen

CLINICAL PEARLS

- Interest in complementary and integrative medicine (CIM) approaches is higher among patients with cancer than in the general population.

- Patients want to discuss CIM approaches with their medical team; however, many find their team members are not receptive or do not have time to engage in such discussions.

- Evidence supports the use of massage to help relieve pain, anxiety, constipation, and nausea and to improve overall quality of life.

INTRODUCTION AND DEFINITIONS

- The terms *integrative*, *alternative*, and *complementary* are not interchangeable:

  - *Integrative Medicine* is an approach to patient care that blends complementary health methods and lifestyle medicine with conventional medicine in a deliberate manner that is personalized, evidence informed, and safe.
  - *Alternative* medicine refers to use of nonconventional approaches in place of conventional medicine.
  - *Complementary* medicine refers to the use of nonconventional approaches together with conventional medicine.
  - *Integrative oncology* refers to the application of integrative medicine to the care of patients with cancer and their caregivers.

- Complementary health approaches (Table 8.1), as defined by the National Center for Complementary and Integrative Health, encompass specialties including natural products (herbs, vitamins and minerals, probiotics), mind and body practices (yoga, meditation, massage, acupuncture), and other systems of care (traditional Chinese medicine, naturopathy).

TABLE 8.1 Complementary Health Approaches[a]

Categories	Examples
Natural products	Herbal medicines (botanicals)
	Vitamins and minerals
	Probiotics
Mind and body practices	Meditation
	Yoga
	Acupuncture
	Qigong and Tai Chi
	Massage therapy
	Chiropractic and osteopathic manipulation
	Acupuncture
	Relaxation techniques (breathing exercises, guided imagery, progressive muscle relaxation)
	Healing touch
	Hypnotherapy
	Movement therapies (Feldenkrais method, Pilates)
Other complementary health approaches	Traditional healers
	Whole medical systems
	■ Ayurvedic medicine
	■ Traditional Chinese medicine
	■ Homeopathy
	■ Naturopathy

[a]As defined by the National Center for Complementary and Integrative Health.

■ In a national survey of adults in the United States, the most commonly used complementary health approaches in the previous year included natural products (17.7%), deep breathing (10.9%) and yoga, Tai Chi, or qigong (10.1%).

INTEGRATIVE CARE PLANNING IN CANCER SURVIVORSHIP: PATIENT–CLINICIAN COMMUNICATION

• Interest in CIM approaches is higher among patients with cancer than in the general population:

  ■ As many as 38% of Americans use CIM approaches, and as many as 68% of these people are patients who have had cancer.
  ■ Patients seeking CIM approaches do so with the goal to experience relief of cancer or cancer treatment-related side effects and better quality of life; they hope these approaches can improve treatment outcomes and decrease recurrence risk, support the immune system, and/or treat other chronic health conditions.

TABLE 8.2 Integrative Medicine Patient Care Talking Points

Perform a baseline assessment that covers lifestyle factors and symptoms or administer a quality-of-life survey.

Create a comfortable environment that encourages open communication. Pay attention to your own and the patient's (and caregiver's) verbal and nonverbal cues.

Assess patient/caregiver goals and level of understanding regarding complementary integrative medicine.

Ask about

- Current or prior experience with and interest in complementary integrative approaches including natural product use and engagement in mind–body practices
- Lifestyle assessment including a review of diet, level of physical activity, stress management, and sleep hygiene

Provide education and evidence-informed recommendations regarding topics of interest as appropriate.

Ask about

- Past or present resources used to learn about complementary integrative medicine (e.g., Internet, textbook, and complementary health provider)

Assess for understanding regarding education provided and topics reviewed.

Provide education materials, relevant references, and resources and a summary of recommendations as part of an integrative care plan.

Encourage follow-up as appropriate to review integrative care plan progress and address new questions that may develop.

Communicate the integrative care plan with a multidisciplinary team of providers including an oncology care team and complementary health practitioners.

Source: Adapted from Lopez G, Mao JJ, Cohen L. Integrative oncology. *Med Clin North Am.* 2017;101(5):977–985.

- Patient–clinician communication regarding CIM (Table 8.2):

  - Patients may make decisions regarding their use of CIM approaches after using unreliable resources; the Internet, media, or clinicians may not provide adequate information.
  - Concerns arise when patients do not communicate their use of CIM approaches to their oncology care team.
  - Patients want to discuss CIM approaches with their medical team; however, many find their team members are not receptive or do not have time to engage in such discussions.
  - It is important to create an environment that encourages open communication regarding interest or use of CIM approaches.
  - It is best to engage in conversations regarding CIM use early on to identify concerns about safety, toxicity, or herb–drug interactions that may adversely influence treatment outcomes.

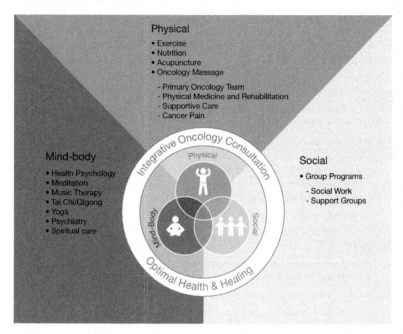

FIGURE 8.1 Integrative oncology model.

- Incorporating questions about interest or use of CIM approaches as part of the standard clinical encounter can help to encourage open communication and strengthen the therapeutic alliance.
- To better address patient needs in the area of integrative oncology, an increasing number of centers now offer formal integrative oncology consultation services.
- Integrative oncology model:
  - The MD Anderson Cancer Center Integrative Medicine Program offers formal integrative oncology consultations with a physician in the Integrative Medicine Center.
  - From diagnosis through survivorship, the integrative oncology model can guide the development of a patient's integrative care plan as part of an integrative oncology consultation (Figure 8.1).
  - The focus on physical health, social health, and mind body/psychosocial health as essential components of patient care is based on the biopsychosocial model as described by George Engel in 1977.
  - An integrative care plan involves:
    o An initial assessment including patient-reported outcome measures of integrative medicine interests, self-reported symptoms, and quality of life

o A review of current or prior experience with and interest in complementary integrative approaches including natural product use, special diets, and engagement in mind and body practices
o A lifestyle assessment including a review of diet, level of physical activity, stress management, and sleep hygiene
o Education and referral to CIM clinicians/therapists (oncology massage, acupuncture, music therapy, physical therapy, nutrition, health psychology, and mind–body approaches such as mediation or yoga) as appropriate

SAFETY CONCERNS

- Mind and body approaches:

  - Concerns exist regarding the safety of engaging in mind and body approaches without proper guidance.
  - Evidence-informed guidance regarding use of mind and body approaches can include safety precautions with modifications based on individual needs.
  - With adequate knowledge of safety precautions, mind and body approaches such as oncology massage, acupuncture, meditation, Tai Chi/qigong, and yoga can be used safely during care.
  - Conditions necessitating modification may include the following:
    o Neutropenia, thrombocytopenia, or fever
    o Anticoagulant use or deep venous thrombosis
    o Presence of metastatic disease or compression fracture
    o Recent surgery, chemotherapy, or radiation treatment
    o Mental status changes, delirium, or involuntary movements
    o Fall risk for movement-based approaches such as yoga, Tai Chi, and qigong

- Natural products, herbs, and supplements: Levels of evidence:

  - May range from opinions and case reports to systematic reviews
  - A thorough understanding of evidence and peer-reviewed literature is important when making a decision regarding natural product, herb, or supplement use during or after cancer care
  - Misinterpretation of available data may lead to misrepresentation of beneficial versus harmful effects of a particular product

- Natural products, herbs, and supplements: Quality control standards:

  - Concerns exist regarding the quality, claims, and labeling of herbal and vitamin supplements available for purchase through a variety of venues including the Internet and health food stores.
  - Studies have identified quality control problems such as:
    o Inaccurate amount of advertised product
    o Mislabeling including absence of the advertised product, product substitution, or use of fillers
    o Contaminants, including heavy metals such as lead or mercury

- ■ Some organizations offer independent review of supplements to assess quality standards of a specific product
- Natural products, herbs, and supplements: Metabolic and treatment interactions:
  - ■ Concerns exist surrounding the uninformed use of vitamins, minerals, and herbal supplements during and after cancer care.
  - ■ Use of vitamin or mineral supplements is best limited to situations in which there is a known or anticipated deficiency, either from a pre-existing condition or as a result of cancer treatments.
  - ■ Alterations in drug metabolism secondary to drug–herb–supplement interactions may interfere with treatment efficacy or contribute to increased toxicity.
  - ■ Concerns regarding use of antioxidant supplements include potential to interfere with chemotherapy or radiation treatment efficacy.
- Natural products, herbs, and supplements: Organ toxicity:
  - ■ Herbal products are associated with direct organ toxicities, including potential for harm to the liver (green tea extract and valerian) or kidneys (bladder wrack and licorice).
  - ■ Certain herbal products (ginkgo biloba, saw palmetto, fish oil, and garlic extracts) may contribute to increased bleeding risk in the setting of surgery or concurrent anticoagulant use.
  - ■ Unpredictable immunomodulatory effects from products such as mushroom extracts and astragalus can be of concern for patients receiving immunosuppressants or other immune-based cancer therapies.
  - ■ A thorough review of herbal product interest or use is important to prevent toxicity or to discontinue products that may contribute to observed organ injury.
- Natural products, herbs, and supplements: Cancer promotion:
  - ■ Plant-based products that contain phytoestrogens may present a safety concern in patients with hormone-sensitive cancers. Black cohosh, chasteberry, evening primrose oil, and red clover are examples.
  - ■ Although soy products contain phytoestrogens, consumption of soy as a food, not a supplement, is not contraindicated and may be included as part of a healthy diet.

COMPLEMENTARY HEALTH APPROACHES: AN EVIDENCE-BASED APPROACH

- As part of developing an integrative care plan, emphasis is placed on using an evidence-informed approach when considering CIM approaches.
- Evidence supports the use of CIM approaches such as acupuncture, oncology massage, and mind–body practices (yoga, Tai Chi/qigong, meditation) in oncology care.

- Acupuncture:
  - Background:
    - According to the National Cancer Institute, acupuncture is defined as "the application of stimulation such as needling, moxibustion, cupping, and acupressure on specific sites of the body known as acupuncture points."
    - Acupuncture has been practiced in China and other Asian countries for thousands of years and in the United States for approximately 200 years.
    - Acupuncture needles were approved by the U.S. Food and Drug Administration as a medical device in 1996.
    - One or more symptoms can be addressed during a single treatment as part of an overall treatment plan.
  - Clinical studies:
    - Clinical research supports the use of acupuncture to help provide relief for a wide variety of symptoms.
    - The strongest evidence favors use of acupuncture to manage pain and chemotherapy- and anesthesia-induced nausea and vomiting.
    - Although additional research is needed, acupuncture may help manage symptoms of chemotherapy-induced peripheral neuropathy, radiation-induced xerostomia, fatigue, hot flashes, postsurgical ileus, anxiety/mood disorders, and sleep disturbances.
    - Pilot studies demonstrated that acupuncture was safe and potentially effective in reducing swelling and improving symptoms in patients with upper- and lower-extremity edema.
  - Safety:
    - A clinician with appropriate training and licensure must administer treatment.
    - Acupuncture has an excellent safety profile, posing low risk for complications that include minimal pain and bruising and possible fainting.
    - Appropriate precautions are needed for patients with immunodeficiency (low neutrophil count), compromised skin integrity, or increased bleeding risk (low platelet count or anticoagulant use).
    - Electroacupuncture may be contraindicated for patients with pacemakers or other implanted devices.
- Oncology massage:
  - Background:
    - Oncology massage refers to the modification of massage technique to address the unique needs of patients with cancer.
  - Clinical studies:
    - Evidence supports the use of massage to help relieve pain, anxiety, constipation, and nausea and to improve overall quality of life.
    - Preliminary evidence in the form of a case report suggests potential benefit for relief of chemotherapy-induced peripheral neuropathy.

- o More research is needed to better understand the type, duration, and frequency of massage treatments best suited to help manage specific symptoms or sets of symptoms.
- Safety:
  - o Massage is safe when provided by clinicians with appropriate training and licensure.
  - o Patients with cancer may need modifications such as site restrictions or changes in level of pressure, depth, or positioning.
  - o Site restrictions may involve recent surgery, lymphedema, deep venous thrombosis, compression fracture, or implanted medical devices.
  - o Precautions also are needed for patients with immunodeficiency (e.g., neutropenia) or those at increased bleeding risk attributable to thrombocytopenia or anticoagulant use.

- Mind and body practices:

  - Background:
    - o Mind and body practices can help support cancer survivors through positive effects on physical and psychosocial health.
    - o Movement-based mind and body practices include yoga, Tai Chi, and qigong.
    - o Additional practices include hypnosis; visual imagery; biofeedback; meditation; cognitive behavioral therapy; and expressive arts such as music, art making, and dance.
  - Clinical studies:
    - o Physical health benefits may include relief of symptoms including pain, nausea, sleep disturbance, and physical function.
    - o Psychosocial health benefits may include relief of anxiety, depressive symptoms, and stress and improved psychosocial factors such as social integration, spirituality, and meaning-making.
    - o Mind and body practices help improve multiple aspects of physical and psychosocial health.

- Safety:

  - Mind–body practices have an excellent safety profile, especially when offered through practitioners with experience working with patients with cancer.
  - Open communication between the patient, healthcare team, and mind–body practitioner can help increase safety through discussion about needs for modifications based on treatment history.

RELIABLE RESOURCES

- Patients, CIM providers, and conventional healthcare providers must make informed decisions regarding CIM based on the latest evidence from reliable resources.
- Reliable online resources for CIM use are featured in Table 8.3.

TABLE 8.3 Recommended Integrative Medicine Internet Resources

University of Texas MD Anderson Cancer Center, Integrative Medicine Program	www.mdanderson.org/integrativemedcenter
Memorial Sloan Kettering Cancer Center	www.mskcc.org/cancer-care/treatments/symptom-management/integrative-medicine/herbs
National Center for Complementary and Integrative Health	www.nccih.nih.gov
National Cancer Institute Office of Cancer Complementary and Alternative Medicine	https://cam.cancer.gov
NCI PDQ Cancer Information Summaries: Integrative, Alternative, and Complementary Therapies	www.cancer.gov/publications/pdq/information-summaries/cam
American Institute for Cancer Research	www.aicr.org
Society for Integrative Oncology	www.integrativeonc.org
Natural Medicines	www.naturalmedicines.com

- An increasing number of academic medical centers offer CIM consultations or services as part of formal integrative medicine programs.
- The goal is to provide onsite expertise to help patients and conventional providers develop a safe, evidence-informed integrative care plan from diagnosis through survivorship.

RECOMMENDED READINGS

Archie P, Bruera E, Cohen L. Music-based interventions in palliative cancer care: a review of quantitative studies and neurobiological literature. *Support Care Cancer.* 2013;21(9):2609–2624.

Bairati I, Meyer F, Gélinas M, et al. Randomized trial of antioxidant vitamins to prevent acute adverse effects of radiation therapy in head and neck cancer patients. *J Clin Oncol.* 2005;23(24):5805–5813.

Bauml JM, Chokshi S, Schapira MM, et al. Do attitudes and beliefs regarding complementary and alternative medicine impact its use among patients with cancer? A cross-sectional survey. *Cancer.* 2015;121(14):2431–2438.

Bower JE, Woolery A, Sternlieb B, et al. Yoga for cancer patients and survivors. *Cancer Control.* 2005;12(3):165.

Cassileth BR, Vickers AJ. Massage therapy for symptom control: outcome study at a major cancer center. *J Pain Symptom Manage.* 2004;28(3):244–249.

Chaoul A, Milbury K, Sood AK, et al. Mind-body practices in cancer care. *Curr Oncol Rep.* 2014;16(12):417.

Clarke TC, Black LI, Stussman BJ, et al. Trends in the use of complementary health approaches among adults: United States, 2002–2012. *Natl Health Stat Report.* 2015(79):1.

Courneya KS, McKenzie DC, Mackey JR, et al. Effects of exercise dose and type during breast cancer chemotherapy: multicenter randomized trial. *J Natl Cancer Inst.* 2013;105(23):1821–1832.

Courneya KS, Sellar CM, Stevinson C, et al. Randomized controlled trial of the effects of aerobic exercise on physical functioning and quality of life in lymphoma patients. *J Clin Oncol.* 2009;27(27):4605–4612.

Engel GL. The need for a new medical model: a challenge for biomedicine. *Science.* 1977;196(4286):129–136.

Greenlee H, Balneaves LG, Carlson LE, et al. Clinical practice guidelines on the use of integrative therapies as supportive care in patients treated for breast cancer. *J Natl Cancer Inst Monogr.* 2014;2014(50):346–358.

Kushi LH, Doyle C, McCullough M, et al. American Cancer Society guidelines on nutrition and physical activity for cancer prevention. *CA Cancer J Clin.* 2012;62(1):30–67.

Lawenda BD, Kelly KM, Ladas EJ, et al. Should supplemental antioxidant administration be avoided during chemotherapy and radiation therapy? *J Natl Cancer Inst.* 2008;100(11):773–783.

Lopez G, Mao JJ, Cohen L. Integrative oncology. *Med Clin North Am.* 2017;101(5):977–985.

Lopez G, McQuade J, Cohen L, et al. Integrative oncology physician consultations at a comprehensive cancer center: analysis of demographic, clinical and patient reported outcomes. *J Cancer.* 2017;8(3):395.

Meyerhardt JA, Niedzwiecki D, Hollis D, et al. Association of dietary patterns with cancer recurrence and survival in patients with stage III colon cancer. *JAMA.* 2007;298(7):754–764.

National Cancer Institute. Acupuncture (PDQ)-Health Professional Version. Available at: https://www.cancer.gov/about-cancer/treatment/cam/hp/acupuncture-pdq. Updated October 20, 2016.

National Center for Complementary and Integrative Health. Complementary, alternative, or intergrative health: what's in a name? Updated June 28, 2016. Available at: https://nccih.nih.gov/health/integrative-health

Navarro VJ, Khan I, Björnsson E, et al. Liver injury from herbal and dietary supplements. *Hepatology.* 2017;65(1):363–373.

Newmaster SG, Grguric M, Shanmughanandhan D, et al. DNA barcoding detects contamination and substitution in North American herbal products. *BMC Med.* 2013;11(1):222.

Richardson MA, Sanders T, Palmer JL, et al. Complementary/alternative medicine use in a comprehensive cancer center and the implications for oncology. *J Clin Oncol.* 2000;18(13):2505–2514.

Russell NC, Sumler S-S, Beinhorn CM, et al. Role of massage therapy in cancer care. *J Altern Complement Med.* 2008;14(2):209–214.

9

Childhood Cancer Survivors

Joann L. Ater
Angela Yarbrough

CLINICAL PEARLS

- Because of the large number of different cancers that occur during childhood, risk assessment for various late effects is based on actual treatments rather than the cancer diagnosis.

- Surveillance for primary cancer usually is not the focus of a childhood cancer survivorship clinic if a patient has been treatment free for more than 5 years; however, late recurrences can happen, especially for patients who have had sarcomas and central nervous system tumors.

- Fertility information is cited as an unmet need among young adult cancer survivors.

EPIDEMIOLOGY AND CARE OF CHILDHOOD CANCER SURVIVORS

- Background and overview of childhood cancer:

  - Children and adolescents can have many different types of cancers. The most common cancers are acute leukemia, brain tumors, lymphomas, and a variety of embryonal solid tumors and sarcomas.
  - Overall 5-year survival for children with a cancer diagnosis before age 20 years is now higher than 80%.
  - Childhood cancer is relatively uncommon, with about 16,600 new cases per year in the United States. One in 300 children has a chance of developing cancer before reaching 20 years of age.
  - An estimated 320,000 childhood cancer survivors are living in the United States, and this number is increasing. About 75% of these survivors are now adults.
  - Long-term side effects of childhood cancer and treatments are common and can appear many years into adulthood.
  - When evaluating illnesses and symptoms in adult survivors of childhood cancer, previous treatments for cancer always should be considered.

- Overview of childhood cancer types:

  - Embryonal cancers such as neuroblastoma (malignancy of the sympathetic ganglia and adrenal medulla), Wilms tumor of the kidney, retinoblastoma, and primitive neuroectodermal tumors of the central nervous system (CNS) and soft tissues occur in early childhood with peak incidence before 2 years of age. Acute lymphoid leukemia, non-Hodgkin's lymphoma, and glioma occur with peak incidence at around 4 years of age. Other cancers such as soft-tissue and bone sarcomas (osteosarcoma, Ewing sarcoma, and rhabdomyosarcoma), Hodgkin disease, testicular cancer, and ovarian cancer are more common in adolescents and young adults.

  - Prognosis is related to the specific cancer diagnosis, stage, age at diagnosis, and biological factors including specific mutations within the tumor that results in different rates of cure. Based on these findings, most types of childhood cancers are associated with defined risk groups depending upon odds of survival (low risk, average risk, high risk, and very high risk).

  - Late effects of treatment are related to the specific chemotherapy and radiation field, age at treatment, complications during treatment, total cumulative doses of the different chemotherapeutic agents, and any genetic predisposition a child may have.

- Clinical tools to guide care for childhood cancer survivors:

  - Because of the large number of different cancers that occur during childhood, risk assessment for various late effects is based on actual treatments rather than the cancer diagnosis.

  - The late effects of radiation to different areas of the body and specific chemotherapeutic agents for patients treated at younger than 21 years of age are detailed by the Children's Oncology Group (COG) at www.survivorshipguidelines.org. These evidence-based recommendations are considered the national standard for survivorship care in children. The recommendations are available to the public but they are quite detailed, and knowledge of specific chemotherapy drugs and doses is necessary. This chapter highlights the most important recommendations and simplifies when possible.

  - Eligibility for childhood cancer survivor clinics varies by institution. Most institutions require that a patient be off of therapy for at least 2 years and not have progressive disease. Patients enter the Childhood Cancer Survivor Study, a national study funded by the National Cancer Institute, when they are 5 years from diagnosis. Consequently, definitions for clinics and research may be different. Some childhood cancer survivor clinics in childrens' hospitals follow patients until they are 21 years of age and then transfer them to an adult survivorship clinic or to the community. Other clinics at major cancer centers such as MD Anderson follow patients treated as children regardless of age. Recommendations for patients treated as children and those treated as adults differ because of age-specific late effects.

- Components of a typical evaluation in a childhood cancer survivorship clinic:

  - All patients should undergo a complete age-appropriate history and physical examination.

- The history should detail the cancer diagnosis, stage if appropriate, age at treatment, and major complications during treatment. If available, the specific chemotherapy drugs and dose and location of radiation are important to determine recommended evaluations and diagnostic tests using the online COG survivorship guidelines. Some patients who are seen in childhood cancer survivor clinics may have an end-of-treatment summary and Passport for Care that outlines their treatment and recommendations for follow-up. Clinic notes from the treating center also may describe treatment and recommended follow-up. If notes are not available, the patient and/or their parents may know this information. Even if exact information is not available, this chapter provides general recommendations based on the cancer diagnosis and most common treatments.
- The history also should include details about growth and development, school performance, anxiety, and other psychosocial issues. Information about diet and exercise habits can be helpful to promote a healthy lifestyle.
- The physical examination should be complete and age appropriate and include height, weight, body mass index or percentage for age (for children younger than 18 years), blood pressure, and Tanner stage of development. Patients treated for CNS tumors, who have had cranial radiation, or are now experiencing symptoms also should have a neurological examination. Special attention should be paid to the original tumor site or sites.
- Laboratory tests and imaging are determined by specific treatments and risks.
- Simplified information according to cancer diagnosis is shown in Table 9.1.

DISEASE SURVEILLANCE

- Surveillance for primary cancer usually is not the focus of a childhood cancer survivorship clinic if a patient has been treatment free for more than 5 years; however, late recurrences can happen, especially for patients who have had sarcomas and CNS tumors. Surveillance for primary cancer is very tumor and protocol specific. Children transferred to a survivorship clinic at fewer than 5 years off treatment usually continue imaging depending upon the primary cancer diagnosis, location, and risk for metastasis. Also, surveillance may be prolonged if a patient is at particularly high risk for recurrence based on tumor pathology, history of metastatic disease, or previous recurrence with subsequent treatment. General guidelines are shown in Table 9.2.

- Childhood cancer survivors also are at risk for subsequent neoplasms, as detailed in Table 9.3. Recommended tests and screenings are detailed. The most important components of surveillance for subsequent neoplasms are a complete history and physical examination and imaging based on symptoms and findings.

- All patients should have a complete age-appropriate history and physical examination with attention to any specific symptoms and the previous cancer site.

- Diagnostic testing:

  - General surveillance guidelines for different types of childhood cancer are shown in Table 9.1.

TABLE 9.1 Monitoring for Late Effects Based on Diagnosis When Detailed Treatment Information Is Not Available[a]

Cancer Diagnosis	Primary Site	Laboratory Tests and Frequency	Diagnostic Tests and Frequency
General for all survivors of childhood cancer	Any	Complete blood count, urinalysis, electrolytes, magnesium, calcium, phosphorus, blood urea nitrogen, creatinine, fasting glucose, bilirubin, ALT yearly	Annual history and physical examination with blood pressure, height, weight, and body mass index (monitor for obesity)
Additional Tests for Specific Diagnoses			
Acute leukemia (ALL and AML)	Bone marrow CNS, testes, ovary	Thyroxine, thyroid-stimulating hormone, follicle-stimulating hormone, luteinizing hormone, estrogen/testosterone if cranial radiation; fasting lipid panel yearly; sperm count if patient wishes	Annual neurologic examination if cranial radiation; eye examination for cataracts; echocardiogram or electrocardiogram following guidelines; bone density at 18 y and 2–3 y after if abnormal findings; neuropsychological evaluation if clinically indicated
CNS tumors	Brain and spinal cord	Same as leukemia	Same as ALL/AML; neuropsychological evaluation repeated every 3–5 y after treatment completion or if school or employment issues arise; audiogram at baseline and every 5 y thereafter

(continued)

TABLE 9.1 Monitoring for Late Effects Based on Diagnosis When Detailed Treatment Information Is Not Available[a] (*continued*)

Cancer Diagnosis	Primary Site	Laboratory Tests and Frequency	Diagnostic Tests and Frequency
Hodgkin/non-Hodgkin's lymphoma	Neck and chest Abdomen and pelvis	Same as leukemia	Chest x-ray, pulmonary function tests at baseline and every 3 y thereafter (more often if the patient received carmustine, lomustine, or bleomycin), echocardiogram and electrocardiogram per guidelines, breast screening per Table 9.3
Wilms tumor, neuroblastoma, rhabdomyosarcoma, germ cell tumors, hepatoblastoma, other solid tumors	Head, neck, chest	Same as leukemia	Same as Hodgkin disease for neck/chest, plus audiogram 5 y after treatment completion and as necessary if the patient received cisplatin
	Abdomen, pelvis		Same as chest, plus colonoscopy per Table 9.3
Ewing sarcoma and osteosarcoma	Long bones, chest, pelvis	Same as leukemia	X-ray of limb yearly Same as Hodgkin disease for neck/chest

ALL, acute myeloid leukemia; ALT, alanine aminotransferase; AML, acute myeloid leukemia; CNS, central nervous system.

[a]These guidelines are most appropriate for patients with a history of chemotherapy and/or radiotherapy.

Source: Modified from Ater JL. Adult survivorship of pediatric cancers. In: Foxhall LE, Rodriguez MA, eds. *Advances in Cancer Survivorship Management*. New York, NY: Springer; 2015:41–56. By permission from Springer Nature.

TABLE 9.2 Off-Therapy Follow-Up Surveillance for Childhood Cancer Survivors

Cancer Type	Year 1 (Test/interval [see key])	Year 2	Year 3	Year 4	Year 5	More Than 5 Years
Leukemia (ALL, AML)	1, 3 Every 4 wk	1, 3 Every 2 mo	1, 3 Every 3 mo	1, 3 Every 6 mo	1, 3 Every 6–12 mo	1, 3 yearly
Lymphoma, Hodgkin disease	1, 3, 15, 6 Every 3 mo	1, 3, 15, 6 Every 6 mo	1, 3, 15, 6 Every 6 mo	1, 3, 15, 6 Every 6 mo	1, 3, 15 yearly	1, 3, 15 yearly
Glioma (high and low grade)	1, 2, 7 Every 3 mo	1, 2, 7 Every 3 mo	1, 2, 7 Every 4 mo	1, 2, 7 Every 6 mo	1, 2, 7 Every 6 mo	1, 2 yearly; 7 yearly up to 10 y
Medulloblastoma/ ependymoma	1, 2, 7, 8 Every 3 mo	1, 2, 7, 8 Every 4 mo	1, 2, 7, 8 Every 6 mo	1, 2, 7 Every year; 8 if previous abnormal findings	1, 2, 7 Every year; 8 if previous abnormal findings	1, 2, 7 Every year; 8 if previous abnormal findings
Bone sarcomas (Ewing, osteosarcoma)	1, 5, 6 Every 3 mo	1, 5, 6 Every 3 mo	1, 5, 6 Every 3 mo	1, 4, or 5, 6 Every 6 mo	1, 4, or 5, 6 Every year	1, 4, 12 Yearly up to 10 y
Soft-tissue sarcomas	1, 4 or 5, 6 Every 3 mo	1, 4 or 5, 6 Every 4 mo	1, 4 or 5, 6 Every 4 mo	1, 5, 6 Every 6 mo	1, 5, 6 Every 6 mo	1 Yearly
Renal tumors	1, 5, 6 Every 3 mo	1, 5, 6, or 9 Every 3 mo	1, 4, 9 Every 6 mo	1, 4, 9 Every 6 mo	1, 4, 9 Every 6 mo	1 Yearly; 4, 9 as indicated
Neuroblastoma	1, 6, 10, 13, 14 Every 3 mo	1, 6, 10, 13, 14 Every 6 mo	1, 6, 10, 13, 14 Every 6 mo	1, 6, 10 Every 6 mo	1, 6, 10 Every 6 mo	1, 10 Yearly
Hepatoblastoma	1, 11 Every 2 mo	1, 11 Every 3 mo	1, 11 Every 3 mo	1, 11 Every 4 mo	1, 11 Every 6 mo	1, 11 Yearly
Germ cell tumors	1, 4, 6, 11 Every 3 mo	1, 11 Every 3 mo; 4, 6 every 6 mo	1, 11 Yearly	1, 11 Yearly	1, 11 Yearly	1, 11 Yearly

(continued)

TABLE 9.2 Off-Therapy Follow-Up Surveillance for Childhood Cancer Survivors (*continued*)

Note: These are generally recommended tests for surveillance. If a patient is enrolled on a protocol, the protocol-specific follow-up should be used. If symptoms appear, tests should be done sooner. If results are abnormal, the patient should be referred back to their primary pediatric oncologist for evaluation.

Surveillance test key

1. History and physical examination
2. Neurological examination
3. CBC with differential and platelets
4. Chest x-ray
5. Chest CT
6. Imaging of primary tumor site with CT or MRI
7. Brain MRI with and without gadolinium
8. Spine MRI with gadolinium
9. Abdominal ultrasound
10. Urinary spot HVA and VMA in mg/gm creatinine
11. Serum alpha-fetoprotein, beta HCG for germ cell tumors; alpha-fetoprotein for hepatoblastoma
12. Plain x-ray of primary bone tumor site
13. MIBG scan for neuroblastoma
14. Bone scan only if positive for bone metastases at diagnosis and non-MIBG avid neuroblastoma
15. Erythrocyte sedimentation rate

ALL, acute lymphoblastic leukemia; AML, acute myeloid leukemia; CBC, complete blood count; HCG, human chorionic gonadotropin; HVA, homovanillic acid; MIBG, metaiodobenzylguanidine; VMA, vanillylmandelic acid.

TABLE 9.3 Modified Screening Recommendations for Childhood Cancer Survivors

Second Malignant Neoplasm	Risk Factors	Screening Recommendations
Skin cancer	10%–20% of patients; increased risk in irradiated skin	Annual skin examination by a dermatologist; closer monitoring of irradiated skin and palms and soles
Breast cancer	Risk in women younger than age 30 is elevated 5- to 54-fold depending on radiation dose to thorax	Yearly mammograms or breast MRI 8 y after radiation or at age 25, whichever occurs later for women who had chest radiation
Thyroid cancer	Increased risk with radiation to the head, neck, and chest	H & P, free T4, TSH yearly, thyroid ultrasound every 3–4 y or sooner if nodules are seen on examination
Leukemia (AML/MDS)	Increased risk with alkylating agents, topoisomerase inhibitors	H & P, annual CBC with differential and platelet count (highest risk first 5 y after exposure)
Brain tumors (glioma and meningioma)	Increased risk with cranial radiation; younger age higher risk; cranial radiation given in setting of brain tumor, ALL, and some head and neck sarcomas	Latency period 9–10 y after radiation; monitor with H & P with neurological examination yearly and MRI of brain if indicated by H & P symptoms
Other carcinomas	Can occur in patients with and without radiation therapy	Latency period 5–30 y, median 15 y; yearly H & P; if abdominal radiation, colon cancer screening with colonoscopy every 10 y beginning 15 y after treatment or at age 35, whichever is later

AML, acute myeloid leukemia; CBC, complete blood count; H & P, history and physical; MDS, myelodysplastic syndromes; TSH, thyroid-stimulating hormone.

Source: Modified from Ater JL. Adult survivorship of pediatric cancers. In: Foxhall LE, Rodriguez MA, eds. *Advances in Cancer Survivorship Management*. New York, NY: Springer; 2015:41–56. By permission from Springer Nature.

■ Children and adolescents with genetic cancer predisposition syndromes are at additional risks for secondary cancers. These syndromes include neurofibromatosis types 1 and 2, retinoblastoma with RB1 constitutional mutations, and Li-Fraumeni syndrome (p53 mutation). These patients should attend a genetics consultation about risks and preferably be followed in a specialized clinic that can plan appropriate surveillance.

MONITORING FOR LATE EFFECTS

- Risk-based monitoring is based on specific treatments:

  - For details about monitoring for late effects in childhood cancer survivors, please see www.survivorshipguidelines.org.
  - Table 9.1 outlines general recommendations based on cancer diagnosis if exact treatment information is easily accessible.

- Late effects by system that differ from adult late effects:

  - Growth and development assessment in childhood cancer survivors is an important part of late effects monitoring. Not only should height, weight, body mass index, and growth percentage be monitored, but Tanner staging should be routinely assessed with a thorough physical examination. Growth disturbances may be caused by poor nutrition, growth hormone deficiency, use of glucocorticoids, or other endocrinopathies such as hypothyroidism or hypogonadism. Radiation therapy to the spine also can damage the epiphyses and lead to disproportionate growth and short stature.
  - Endocrine sequelae are highest among patients who receive treatment with radiation therapy and certain chemotherapies and may not be present for many years. Possible endocrinopathies related to treatment include growth hormone deficiency, central hypothyroidism, central adrenal insufficiency, hyperprolactinemia, precocious puberty, hypogonadotropic hypogonadism, being overweight, and obesity. Detailed classifications of high-risk treatment exposure for development of endocrinopathy are shown in Table 9.4. Growth and pubertal development should be monitored every 6 months with an examination.
    - o Growth hormone deficiency is directly related to doses of radiation exposure and inversely related to age of exposure. Clinical presentation may be subtle and may manifest only with a diminished pubertal growth spurt. Insulin-like growth factor should be checked at baseline when receiving radiation therapy and at least annually.
    - o Central hypothyroidism is associated with radiation doses higher than 40 Gy to the hypothalamic axis. This diagnosis may be difficult to establish, particularly when it is mild. Free T4 level should be checked at least annually.
    - o Primary hypothyroidism is caused by direct damage to the thyroid gland by radiation therapy at doses higher than 10 Gy. Thyroid-stimulating hormone should be checked at least annually and every 6 months until a patient progresses through puberty.
    - o Patients who have had more than 40 Gy of radiation to the hypothalamic axis and exposure to exogenous steroids are at higher risk for central adrenal insufficiency. This problem is less common than other endocrinopathies. Random 8 a.m. cortisol levels should be checked annually.
    - o Hyperprolactinemia is associated with radiation doses higher than 50 Gy to the hypothalamic axis. Elevated prolactin levels may cause galactorrhea in females and hypogonadism in either gender. Prolactin level should be tested annually.

TABLE 9.4 Treatment Exposures Posing High Risk for Endocrinopathy

Endocrine Disorder	Therapeutic Exposure
Primary hypothyroidism	Thyroid irradiation exceeding 20 Gy
Central hypothyroidism	Hypothalamic pituitary irradiation with more than 40 Gy
Hyperthyroidism	Thyroid irradiation with more than 40 Gy
Central adrenal insufficiency	Hypothalamic pituitary irradiation with more than 30 Gy
Growth hormone deficiency	Hypothalamic pituitary irradiation with more than 18 Gy
Precocious puberty	Hypothalamic pituitary irradiation with more than 18 Gy
Hyperprolactinemia	Hypothalamic pituitary irradiation with more than 40 Gy
Gonadotropin deficiency	Hypothalamic pituitary irradiation with more than 30 Gy in men and women More than 20 Gy testicular radiation in men

Source: Adapted from the Children's Oncology Group. Long-term follow-up guidelines for survivors of childhood, adolescent, and young adult cancers. 2013. Available at: www.survivorshipguidelines.org

○ Abnormal puberty may include precocious puberty and gonadotropin deficiencies in both boys and girls. Central gonadal dysfunction may occur in males and females receiving more than 30 Gy. Testosterone, luteinizing hormone (LH), and follicle-stimulating hormone (FSH) should be checked annually in males, and estradiol, LH, and FSH should be checked annually in females.

○ Childhood survivors treated with more than 18 Gy of cranial irradiation are at increased risk for obesity, and those exposed to abdominal irradiation or total body irradiation (TBI) are at higher risk for diabetes mellitus. Consider evaluation for other comorbid conditions including dyslipidemia, hypertension, or impaired glucose metabolism if obesity is present.

▪ Cardiotoxicity is a serious late effect of childhood cancer treatment. Anthracycline-based chemotherapy (e.g., doxorubicin, daunorubicin, idarubicin) and radiation to the mediastinum and neck are the most common causes of cardiotoxicity. About 50% of childhood survivors have received anthracyclines. Both early- and late-onset cardiotoxicity can occur:

○ Childhood survivors should undergo routine echocardiogram screening depending upon their age at treatment exposure to anthracyclines and radiation therapy as recommended by the COG's long-term follow-up guidelines.

○ Patients who were treated for lymphoma, Hodgkin's lymphoma, sarcomas, or myeloid leukemia are at highest risk for cardiotoxicity because they receive high doses of anthracycline.

- o Because deterioration in cardiac function can occur many years after treatment, long-term monitoring with echocardiograms is recommended.
- ▪ Cognitive deficits occur in children treated with cranial irradiation, especially whole-brain irradiation. Intrathecal chemotherapy also can contribute to deficits. Cognitive problems may become apparent several years after treatment and usually increase over time:
  - o Children younger than 7 years of age at the time of radiotherapy are at highest risk for cognitive deficits including a decrease in IQ, poor attention, poor memory, and deficits in executive functioning.
  - o Young children treated with TBI also are at risk for decreased cognitive function.
  - o Older children treated with lower doses of radiation (such as doses for CNS prophylaxis for leukemia) also are at risk for cognitive decline later in life.
  - o Survivors of childhood cancer of any age should undergo neuropsychological testing if they are experiencing problems at school or cognitive issues because these issues may be related to treatment.
  - o If neuropsychological testing reveals characteristics of attention deficit disorder (ADD), the child or adolescent should be referred to a pediatric neurologist for treatment.
- ▪ Fertility information is cited as an unmet need among young adult cancer survivors. Education and counseling should address individual fertility risks and alternative methods of family planning such as those provided by the oncofertility service at MD Anderson Cancer Center.

RISK REDUCTION/EARLY DETECTION

- As shown in Table 9.3, breast and colon cancer screening guidelines for adults who received cancer treatment as children are different if a patient has had either chest or abdominal radiation.

- For both girls and boys ages 11 to 25, the human papillomavirus (HPV) vaccine should be recommended to prevent HPV-related cancers.

- Refer all tobacco users to a smoking cessation program.

- A heart-healthy diet and exercise are especially important for childhood cancer survivors to decrease obesity and reduce risk for second cancers in adulthood and to improve cardiovascular health.

- Following relapse and a second cancer, the most common cause of premature morbidity and mortality among childhood cancer survivors is cardiovascular disease at an earlier age than expected.

- For patients who received anthracyclines and/or chest radiation as children, risk for cardiomyopathy and cardiovascular disease increases dramatically (12–32 times) if a patient also has hypertension. Other cardiovascular risk factors such as obesity, type 2 diabetes, and hyperlipidemia increase risk. Controlling these risk factors is essential to help ensure long-term health and is part of survivorship care.

PSYCHOSOCIAL HEALTH AND FUNCTIONING

- The Childhood Cancer Survivor Study revealed that childhood cancer survivors are at higher risk than their sibling controls for anxiety, social withdrawal, educational problems, dysfunctional marital relationships, unemployment or underemployment, and dependent living. Survivors of brain tumors and patients who have had leukemia and cranial radiation are at highest risk for impaired intellectual functioning. These patients also are at increased risk for difficulty obtaining and maintaining medical insurance coverage.

- At MD Anderson's Childhood Cancer Survivor Clinic, the most commonly requested psychosocial services are vocational counseling, neuropsychological testing (because of poor school performance), school intervention (to ensure a child's educational program is appropriate), and referrals to psychology or psychiatry to address anxiety and depression.

- For young adult survivors who are otherwise functioning well, one of the most common concerns is fertility and the ability to have a family. Referral to a fertility specialist can be helpful.

- School and educational issues are especially important, and problems do not end when treatment ends. At survivorship clinic visits, always include questions about school performance during interviews. A child may be entitled to special services at school. Inattention and difficulty concentrating also are fairly common, and treatment may be effective if ADD is diagnosed.

CLINICAL VIGNETTE

MR is a 12-year-old young girl with a history of nonmetastatic group 3 (biopsy) stage II (parameningeal) embryonal rhabdomyosarcoma. She received standard of care chemotherapy consisting of vincristine, dactinomycin, and cyclophosphamide for intermediate risk disease. Given her cranial nerve involvement, the recommendation was made for proton beam radiation. She received a maximum dose of 52 cGy to the pituitary gland.

Questions

1. Which of the following pituitary hormones is most sensitive to the effects of radiation therapy?
   A. Luteininzing hormone
   B. Antidiuretic hormone
   C. TSH

   D. ACTH
   E. Growth hormone

2. Prognosis of childhood cancer is related to which of the following factors
   A. Specific cancer diagnosis
   B. Stage
   C. Age at diagnosis
   D. Biological factors including specific mutations within the tumor
   E. All of the above

3. MR arrives to your clinic as a new patient. What age-appropriate vaccination should this patient receive that will potentially decrease her risk of related cancers?
   A. Influenza vaccine
   B. Human Papilloma vaccine
   C. Meningococcal vaccine
   D. None of the above

4. This patient is at risk for the following endocrinopathies related to radiation therapy
   A. Hyperprolactinemia
   B. Central hypothyroidism
   C. Primary hypothyroidism
   D. All of the above
   E. Only A and B

Answers

1. E
Growth hormone deficiency is directly related to the dose of radiation exposure, and is increased in patients who have received greater than 18 Gy to the hypothalamic pituitary axis. Highest risk factors include younger age at treatment, higher radiation doses, surgery in the suprasellar region, and pre-transplant radiation.

2. E
Prognosis of childhood cancer is related to multiple factors including the specific cancer diagnosis, stage, age at diagnosis, and biological factors including specific genetic mutations within the tumor. Most types of childhood cancers are associated with defined risk groups depending on odds of survival based on the above factors.

3. B
The HPV can cause cervical cancer in women and other less common cancers such as anal, vulvar, vaginal, and oropharyngeal as well. The HPV vaccine is recommended by the Centers for Disease Control in all boys and girls ages 11 to 12 to protect against cancers caused by HPV.

4. E
Patients receiving greater than 40 Gy to the hypothalamic pituitary axis are at an increased risk of developing hyperprolactinemia and central hypothyroidism. Primary hypothyroidism is related to a radiation dose of greater than 10 Gy to the thyroid gland directly.

RECOMMENDED READINGS

Armstrong GT, Kawashima T, Leisenring W, et al. Aging and risk of severe, disabling, life-threatening, and fatal events in the childhood cancer survivor study. *J Clin Oncol.* 2014;32(12):1218–1227. doi:10.1200/JCO.2013.51.1055

Armstrong GT, Oeffinger KC, Chen Y, et al. Modifiable risk factors and major cardiac events among adult survivors of childhood cancer. *J Clin Oncol.* 2013;31(29):3673–3680.

Armstrong GT, Stovall M, Robison LL. Long-term effects of radiation exposure among adult survivors of childhood cancer: results from the Childhood Cancer Survivor Study. *Radiat Res.* 2010;174(6):840–850.

Ater JL. Adult survivorship of pediatric cancers. In: Foxhall LE, Rodriguez MA, eds. *Advances in Cancer Survivorship Management.* New York, NY: Springer; 2015:41–56.

Benedict C, Shuk E, Ford JS. Fertility issues in adolescent and young adult cancer survivors. *J Adolesc Young Adult Oncol.* 2016;5(1):48–57.

Castellino SM, Ullrich NJ, Whelen MJ, et al. Developing interventions for cancer-related cognitive dysfunction in childhood cancer survivors. *J Natl Cancer Inst.* 2014;106(8):1–16. doi:10.1093/jnci/dju186

Children's Oncology Group. Long-term follow-up guidelines for survivors of childhood, adolescent, and young adult cancers. 2013. Available at: www.survivorshipguidelines.org.

Chow EJ, Chen Y, Kremer LC, et al. Individual prediction of heart failure among childhood cancer survivors. *J Clin Oncol.* 2015;33(5):394–402.

Foxhall LE, Rodriguez MA, SpringerLink. *Advances in Cancer Survivorship Management.* 2015 ed. New York, NY: Springer; 2015.

Gianinazzi ME, Rueegg CS, Wengenroth L, et al. Adolescent survivors of childhood cancer: are they vulnerable for psychological distress? *Psychooncology.* 2013;22(9):2051–2058.

Henderson TO, Oeffinger KC, Whitton J, et al. Secondary gastrointestinal cancer in childhood cancer survivors: a cohort study. *Ann Intern Med.* 2012;156(11):757–766.

Lipshultz SE, Cochran TR, Franco VI, et al. Treatment-related cardiotoxicity in survivors of childhood cancer. *Nat Rev Clin Oncol.* 2013;10(12):697–710.

Mariotto AB, Rowland JH, Yabroff KR, et al. Long-term survivors of childhood cancers in the United States. *Cancer Epidemiol Biomarkers Prev.* 2009;18(4):1033–1040.

Moskowitz CS, Chou JF, Wolden SL, et al. Breast cancer after chest radiation therapy for childhood cancer. *J Clin Oncol.* 2014;32(21):2217–2223.

Mostoufi-Moab S, Seidel K, Leisenring WM, et al. Endocrine abnormalities in aging survivors of childhood cancer: a report from the Childhood Cancer Survivor Study. *J Clin Oncol.* 2016;34(27):3240–3247.

Mueller S, Sear K, Hills NK, et al. Risk of first and recurrent stroke in childhood cancer survivors treated with cranial and cervical radiation therapy. *Int J Radiat Oncol Biol Phys.* 2013;86(4):643–648.

Mulder RL, Kremer LCM, Hudson MM, et al. Recommendations for breast cancer surveillance for female survivors of childhood, adolescent, and young adult cancer given chest radiation: a report from the International Late Effects of Childhood Cancer Guideline Harmonization Group. *Lancet Oncol.* 2013;14(13):E621–E629.

Ness KK, Hudson MM, Jones KE, et al. Effect of temporal changes in therapeutic exposure on self-reported health status in childhood cancer survivors. *Ann Intern Med.* 2017;166(2):89–98.

Oeffinger KC, Mertens AC, Sklar CA, et al. Chronic health conditions in adult survivors of childhood cancer. *N Engl J Med.* 2006;355(15):1572–1582.

Ratan R, Ater JL, Reiber AG, et al. Long-term survivorship in adult and pediatric cancer. In: Kantarian HN, Wolf R, eds. *MD Anderson Manual of Medical Oncology.* 3rd ed. Houston, TX: MD Anderson; 2016.

Schwartz CL, Hobbie WL, Constine LS, et al. *Survivors of Childhood and Adolescent Cancer.* 3rd ed. New York, NY: Springer; 2015.

Smith WA, Li CH, Nottage KA, et al. Lifestyle and metabolic syndrome in adult survivors of childhood cancer. *Cancer.* 2014;120(17):2742–2750.

Survivorship Care for Patients With Breast Cancer

Joyce E. Dains
Marita Lazzaro

CLINICAL PEARLS

- An annual diagnostic mammogram for patients with noninvasive ductal carcinoma in situ (DCIS) through Year 5 is recommended. An annual screening mammogram for patients with invasive and noninvasive breast cancer for Years 6 and beyond also is recommended (refer to survivorship algorithms).

- Chronic fatigue during the survivorship period should be evaluated as a condition in and of itself.

- Obesity may become a problem. Attempt to motivate survivors to enter a comprehensive weight loss program that includes dietary and exercise counseling as indicated.

BREAST CANCER EPIDEMIOLOGY AND SURVIVORSHIP CARE

- General background

  - Breast cancer is the most common cancer in the United States among women and the second-leading cause of cancer death after lung cancer.
  - A woman living in the United States has a 12.3% risk or a one in eight lifetime risk for breast cancer; incidence increases with age.
  - About 80% of breast cancers occur sporadically; only 5% to 10% are associated with an inherited germline mutation.
  - Breast cancer incidence is highest among non-Hispanic White women, followed by non-Hispanic Black women and Hispanic women. Incidence is lowest among Asian/Pacific Islander women. However, mortality is highest among non-Hispanic Black women.

■ Factors affecting treatment and survival include stage at diagnosis, histologic subtype, hormone receptor status (estrogen or progesterone positive), human epidermal growth factor receptor 2, and gene expression.

■ The overall 5-year relative survival rate for women with breast cancer has improved during the last three decades because of earlier detection and improvements in treatment.

■ The 5-year, 10-year, and 15-year overall relative survival rates for breast cancer are 89%, 83%, and 78%, respectively.

■ Sixty-one percent of breast cancers are diagnosed at a localized stage.

■ When compared with White women, Black women are less likely to have local-stage breast cancer (53% vs. 62%) and experience lower survival rates within each stage.

• The two most common breast neoplasms

  ■ Invasive ductal carcinoma
    o Incidence
      — Accounts for 80% of all invasive breast cancers
      — There are other subtypes of invasive breast cancer; some are associated with better survival rates than others
    o Survival
      — Survival rates vary by disease stage and subtype
        a. Stage I: 5-year relative survival rate is close to 100%
        b. Stage II: 5-year relative survival rate is about 93%
        c. Stage III: 5-year relative survival rate is about 72%
        d. Metastatic: 5-year relative survival rate is about 22%
  ■ Ductal carcinoma in situ (DCIS)
    o Incidence
      — In situ breast carcinomas account for about 20% of all breast cancers in women; of these, 85% are DCIS
      — Incidence increases with age
      — Overall incidence rates are similar for non-Hispanic White, non-Hispanic Black, and Asian/Pacific Islander women; incidence is lower for Hispanic women and lowest for American Indian/Alaska Native women
    o Mortality
      — Prognostic factors include nuclear grade, histology, lesion size, estrogen receptor status, and comedonecrosis
      — Breast-specific mortality at 10 years is 1.1% and at 20 years is 3.3%; mortality is higher for Black women and women with a diagnosis before age 35
    o Survival
      — 5-year survival is close to 100%

• Clinical tools to guide care of breast cancer survivors

  ■ Algorithm for Survivorship, Invasive Breast Cancer (refer to Figure 10.1).
  ■ Algorithm for Survivorship, Noninvasive Breast Cancer (refer to Figure 10.2).
  ■ Algorithm for Breast Cancer Survivorship, Bone Health (refer to Figure 10.3).
  ■ Refer to Chapter 5 for cervical and colorectal cancer screening algorithms

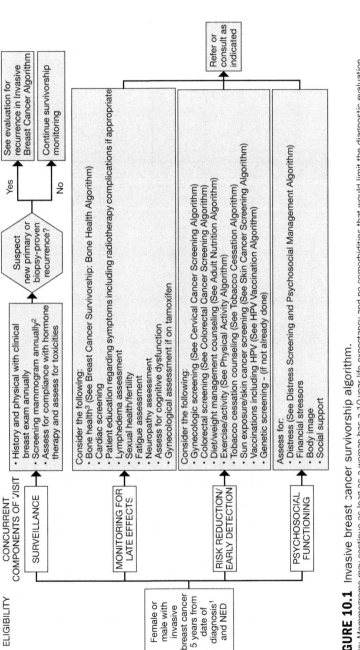

FIGURE 10.1 Invasive breast cancer survivorship algorithm.

Note: Mammograms may continue as long as a woman has a 10-year life expectancy and no comorbidities that would limit the diagnostic evaluation or treatment of any identified problem; NED, no evidence of disease; [1]Completion of all treatment with the exception of hormonal agents; [2]Consider tomosynthesis/3D mammogram; [3]Premenopausal women on hormonal therapy. *Source:* Copyright 2017 The University of Texas MD Anderson Cancer Center.

112

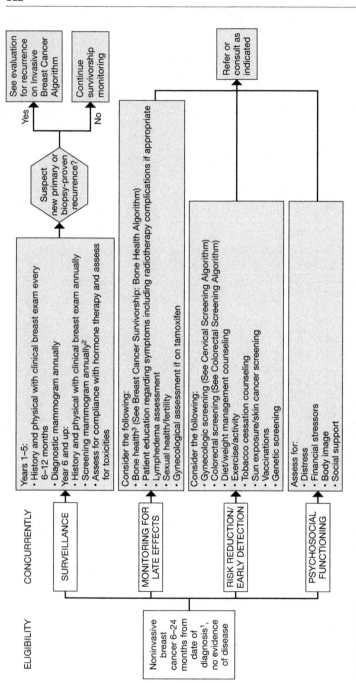

FIGURE 10.2 Noninvasive breast cancer survivorship algorithm.

[1]Completion of all treatment with the exception of hormonal agents; [2]Consider tomosynthesis/3D mammogram; [3]Premenopausal women on tamoxifen or hormonal therapy. *Source:* Copyright 2016 The University of Texas MD Anderson Cancer Center.

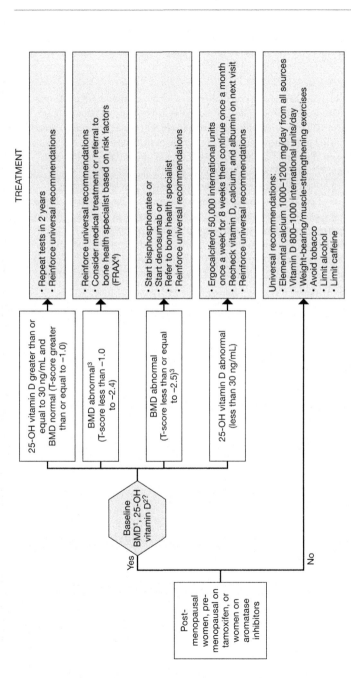

FIGURE 10.3 Bone health breast cancer survivorship algorithm.

[1]BMD, bone mineral density; [2]25-hydroxyvitamin D, also known as 25-hydroxycholecalciferol, calcidiol, or abbreviated as 25-OH vitamin D, the main vitamin D metabolite circulating in plasma; [3]Abnormal BMD (osteopenia, T-score between −1.0 and −2.4; osteoporosis, T-score less than or equal to −2.5); [4]FRAX, WHO Fracture Risk Assessment Tool at www.shef.ac.uk/frax. *Source:* Copyright 2014 The University of Texas MD Anderson Cancer Center.

DISEASE SURVEILLANCE

- Medical history and physical examination

  - Review of systems
    - o Should focus on the most common sites of local recurrence (affected breast and nodal basins) and metastatic disease (bone, lungs, liver, and brain/spinal cord)
    - o Lumps, skin lesions or thickening, nodules or fullness, alteration in appearance
    - o Increasing or persistent focused bone pain (bone metastases)
    - o Pleuritic chest pain, dyspnea, persistent cough (pulmonary metastases)
    - o Abdominal pain, increased abdominal girth, jaundice, early satiety, alteration in consistency or color of stool (liver, ovarian, or gastric metastases)
    - o New or increasing headache, visual changes, nausea, vomiting, dizziness, altered speech and mental status, weakness, changes in sensation, new bowel or bladder incontinence (brain or spinal metastases)
    - o Pelvic pain, irregular or new-onset vaginal bleeding (genitourinary metastases)
    - o Sexuality concerns, dyspareunia, vaginal dryness, premature ovarian failure, return of ovarian function; consider vaginal moisturizers, lubrication, refer for sexuality counseling
  - General examination (refer to Figures 10.1 and 10.2 algorithms)
    - o Complete physical examination annually
    - o Cardiac, pulmonary, and abdominal examinations
    - o Head, eye, ear, nose, and throat examinations as part of a neurologic examination
    - o Lymph node basins (cervical, supraclavicular, infraclavicular, axillary, and inguinal)
    - o Breast examination
      - — Assess for contour change, nipple retraction, skin changes, erythema, thickening, nodules or lumps, vascular changes, and changes in tissue consistency.
      - — Assess the radiation site for radiation-induced atrophy; refer to plastic surgery if severe.
      - — Assess the radiation field for radiation-induced angiosarcoma nodules or purple papules; biopsy may be indicated.
      - — Assess the scar; recurrence may appear as a skin lesion, nodule, or mass along the scar line.
      - — Fat necrosis is a frequent benign occurrence seen in traumatized breast tissue that is attributable to surgery or radiation. This appears as a mass or thickening that can be monitored after a diagnosis is confirmed with imaging/biopsy.
  - Pelvic examination
    - o Routine pelvic examinations are not recommended. Gynecologic assessment is recommended if a patient is taking tamoxifen. Query the survivor regarding vaginal bleeding, spotting, discharge, pain, or a change in abdominal girth (refer to MD Anderson's breast survivorship algorithms [Figures 10.1 and 10.2]; the Endometrial Cancer Screening Algorithm [available at www.mdanderson.org]; and the Cervical Cancer Screening Algorithm [available at www.mdanderson.org]).

- o Query postmenopausal survivors or survivors with premature ovarian failure regarding vaginal dryness, dyspareunia, or postcoital spotting. Cytology/colposcopy may be indicated if postcoital bleeding occurs. Recommend frequent/routine use of vaginal moisturizers and lubricants.
- o Conduct age-appropriate routine screening.
- o Perform a bimanual examination if the survivor reports abdominal pain or a change in abdominal girth.
- o Perform an every-6-month bimanual examination, CA125 lab test, and transvaginal ultrasound if there is a family history of ovarian cancer or BRCA 1/2 mutation (refer to MD Anderson's Ovarian Cancer Screening Algorithm).
- o Routine transvaginal ultrasound and/or endometrial biopsies are not recommended. Testing should be limited to patients with pelvic symptoms or vaginal bleeding/spotting.
- ▪ Musculoskeletal examination (assess for lymphedema, point tenderness on palpation to spine and chest wall)

- Diagnostic testing

- ▪ Laboratory tests
  - o Routine laboratory tests should include a complete blood count (CBC), liver function tests, and carcinoembryonic antigen, and tumor markers (CA 15-3 or CA 27.29) are not recommended
  - o Laboratory tests as indicated to assess concerns
  - o Vitamin D level as indicated for osteoporosis screening or surveillance (refer to Figure 10.3)
  - o Every-6-month CA 125 for BRCA 1/2 mutation carriers
- ▪ Radiologic procedures
  - o Diagnostic mammogram annually for patients with noninvasive DCIS through Year 5; annual screening mammogram for patients with invasive and noninvasive breast cancer for Years 6 and beyond (refer to survivorship algorithms)
  - o MRI as an adjunct to mammography for BRCA 1/2 mutation carriers
  - o Diagnostic imaging evaluation (diagnostic mammogram, ultrasound, MRI) to assess for abnormal clinical or imaging findings on remaining breasts or reconstructed breasts
  - o Ultrasound to assess for abnormal clinical findings at the mastectomy site, chest wall, or nodal basins
- ▪ Special procedures
  - o Bone mineral density testing (refer to Figure 10.3)
  - o Bone scan to address concerns about bone or spinal metastases
  - o Rib series as an adjunct to a bone scan as indicated
  - o Computed tomography scan and/or MRI as indicated to address concerns regarding pulmonary, abdominal, or pelvic metastases
  - o Transvaginal ultrasound and/or endometrial biopsy for vaginal bleeding or spotting, especially for women taking tamoxifen

    o Transvaginal ultrasound with or without CA 125 for pelvic pain, abdominal bloating, or increase in abdominal girth

    o Endometrial biopsy to asses irregular vaginal bleeding or postmenopausal vaginal spotting

- Treatments

  ■ For invasive breast cancer, survivorship is usually 5 years after treatment completion. Hormonal therapy may be extended for an additional 5 years and falls under the realm of survivorship care.

  ■ Tamoxifen or aromatase inhibitor (AI) use as extended therapy for early stage estrogen receptor–positive breast cancer is associated with a decreased overall recurrence rate but not an overall increased survival rate. Anastrozole (Arimidex) reduces the risk for recurrence of early stage breast cancer over tamoxifen in the Arimidex, Tamoxifen, Alone and in Combination Trial. Extended-use options include:

      o Tamoxifen for a total of 10 years of 20 mg orally daily

      o AI with exemestane 25 mg orally daily or anastrozole 1 mg orally daily for a total of 10 years

      o A combination of 5 years of tamoxifen followed by 5 years of an AI

  ■ Risk/benefit analysis should take into account patient age, additional breast cancer risk factors, comorbidities, and risk for adverse effects.

  ■ Tamoxifen is associated with risk for stroke, blood clots, endometrial cancer, and cataracts.

  ■ AIs, which are associated with risk for osteoporosis (refer to Figure 10.3), have a more favorable side effect profile. Bone/joint pain may be controlled with anti-inflammatory medication; consider acupuncture and exercise.

  ■ For noninvasive breast cancer, entrance into survivorship may occur 6 to 24 months after diagnosis. Hormonal treatment for estrogen receptor–positive breast cancer is considered part of survivorship care.

      o Tamoxifen only; 20 mg orally daily for 5 years

MONITORING FOR LATE EFFECTS

- Surgical effects

  ■ Arm lymphedema may occur following mastectomy and axillary node dissection. The change to sentinel node biopsy has reduced this occurrence.

      o Refer to physical therapy for lymphedema evaluation and treatment.

      o There is no weight limit for the arm on the affected side. Rather, rest and elevation is recommended when the arm becomes tired.

      o Lymphedema poses risk for cellulitis. Oral antibiotics may not be as effective in this setting. Close observation to determine resolution or the need for intravenous therapy is necessary.

- o Stewart–Treves syndrome is rare and associated with chronic massive lymph-edema that may lead to lymphangiosarcoma.
  - ▪ Implant encapsulation and calcification may lead to pain, and a referral to plastic surgery may be indicated.
  - ▪ Implant-related anaplastic large B-cell lymphoma is a rare condition that usually appears as fluid around the implant (often an imaging finding). Needle biopsy is indicated for diagnosis.
- Chemotherapy effects

  - ▪ Cardiovascular
    - o Cardiac effects should be monitored by a cardiologist in collaboration with the clinician.
    - o Anthracycline increases dose-dependent risk for congestive heart failure.
    - o Anthracycline-related cardiomyopathy risk increases with age when it is used in conjunction with trastuzumab or mediastinal radiation.
    - o Trastuzumab-related cardiotoxicity is not dose dependent and is usually reversible when treatment ends. Cardiomyopathy is not clinically detectable but can be identified upon further testing.
  - ▪ Neurotoxicity
    - o Chemotherapy neuropathy of the lower extremities and feet and less commonly the hands may be long term.
    - o Pharmaceutical interventions include gabapentin or pregabalin.
    - o Integrative approaches include acupuncture.
    - o Walking, Tai Chi, or water exercise to preserve mobility is recommended.
    - o Cognitive outcome study findings reveal that cognitive decline ranges between 17% and 75%. Prospective studies are conflicting.
    - o Self-perceived cognitive decline is linked to psychological distress and depression.
  - ▪ Chemotherapy-induced ovarian failure
    - o Risk for ovarian failure increases in women older than age 35 who receive cyclophosphamide or anthracycline.
    - o Ovarian failure increases risk for osteoporosis. Patients should be monitored closely with bone mineral density testing and vitamin D levels (refer to Figure 10.3).

- Radiation therapy

  - ▪ Cardiovascular effects have substantially decreased with advances in radiation treatment.
  - ▪ Angiosarcoma is a risk in the radiated field. A solid mass or module should be evaluated with a core biopsy if it is clinically suspicious.
  - ▪ Radiation-induced atrophy, characterized by extreme adhesion to the chest wall and thinning of the skin, is rare but may necessitate plastic surgery intervention.
  - ▪ Adhesions and chronic pain are not uncommon. Physical therapy may provide some success, and nonsteroidal anti-inflammatory medication may relieve pain.

- Hormonal therapies

    - Tamoxifen may increase risk for endometrial cancer or, more rarely, uterine sarcomas.
        - Evaluation of postmenopausal vaginal spotting with endometrial biopsy is indicated.
        - Transvaginal ultrasound can provide uterine/ovarian information prior to biopsy.
        - Abdominal pain, bloating, or an increase in girth should be evaluated with transvaginal ultrasound.
        - Assessing levels of follicle-stimulating hormone, luteinizing hormone, and estradiol may help to establish menopausal status versus return of ovarian function in young women with new-onset vaginal bleeding. Endometrial biopsy should still be considered for patients taking tamoxifen.
        - Tamoxifen increases cataract risk. An annual examination with an ophthalmologist is recommended.
        - Risk for blood clots and stroke is equal to risks associated with hormone replacement therapy. Acute onset of chest pain, lower leg pain, difficulty breathing, and weakness should be evaluated emergently.
    - AI use should be limited to postmenopausal women or women with surgically or chemically induced menopause.
        - AIs are associated with a favorable side effect profile with no increase in vasodilation symptoms.
        - AIs can increase bone loss. Osteoporosis is a risk and its potential necessitates surveillance (refer to Figure 10.3).

- Fatigue

    - Fatigue associated with treatment usually is addressed during the treatment phase. Chronic fatigue during the survivorship period should be evaluated as a condition in and of itself. Referral to a rheumatologist for evaluation may be indicated.

- Menopausal symptoms

    - Whether the result of natural aging or premature ovarian failure, symptoms of menopause are similar.
        - Vasodilation symptoms
            — Hot flashes and night sweats are common early in menopause. Symptoms usually subside or become tolerable within 1 year. Only a handful of women will experience substantial symptoms for longer than 2 to 3 years
            — Symptoms are aggravated by caffeine, stress, and fatigue
            — Regular exercise and weight regulation can control symptoms. Mind/body exercise such as Tai Chi, yoga, or qigong can reduce stress
            — Environmental heat control can help
            — There is no evidence on the safety or efficacy of supplements or herbal preparations for women with history of breast cancer
        - Vaginal dryness/dyspareunia
            — Routine use of vaginal moisturizers is recommended
            — Lubrication with sexual activity is recommended

— Use of vaginal estrogen with an estradiol vaginal ring or a vaginal tablet has a negligible effect on raising circulating estrogen levels above menopause levels. Patients should be counseled and information should be documented regarding risks and benefits. Quality of life versus recurrence risk becomes the issue in the absence of additional contraindications

RISK REDUCTION/EARLY DETECTION

- This section focuses on risk reduction/early detection specific to breast cancer survivors.

  ▪ Refer to Chapter 5 for cancer screening guidelines for colorectal, endometrial, ovarian, liver, lung, and skin cancers.

- Second cancers can be attributed to common risk factors predisposing to both the first and second cancers (e.g., genetic risk, environmental risk) or to treatment-related effects.

  ▪ Breast cancer survivors are at elevated risk for a second primary breast cancer, especially women with a family history of breast cancer.
  ▪ Compared with the general population, breast cancer survivors are at slightly higher risk for a second cancer within the first 10 years after the first diagnosis.
  ▪ Radiation therapy confers a small increased risk for hematologic malignancies, cancer of the esophagus, and angiosarcoma and lung cancer.

- Gynecologic cancer screening

  ▪ Survivors taking tamoxifen are at increased risk for endometrial carcinoma and uterine sarcoma. Vaginal ultrasound is not recommended for screening. Endometrial biopsy should be performed if vaginal bleeding occurs.

- Colorectal cancer screening

  ▪ Screening should follow the guidelines in Chapter 5.

- Diet/weight management

  ▪ Obesity is associated with increased risk for contralateral breast, endometrial, and colorectal secondary primary cancers.

- Exercise/activity

  ▪ There is convincing evidence that physical activity reduces risk for colon cancer; probable evidence for risk reduction in breast and endometrial cancers; and possible evidence for risk reduction in cancers of the prostate, lung, and ovary.
  ▪ Evidence shows that physical activity improves survival among breast cancer survivors.

- Tobacco cessation counseling/lung cancer screening

  ▪ Survivors who have had radiation therapy have slightly higher risk for lung cancer.

- Sun exposure/skin screening

  - Survivors who have had radiation are at a slightly higher risk for angiosarcoma in the treatment field; patients may present with a purple macule or papule that necessitate biopsy.

- Vaccinations

  - Survivors should receive appropriate vaccinations based on their age and medical condition as per standard practice.

- Genetic counseling

  - Women at high risk for familial breast cancer syndromes should be referred for genetic counseling in accordance with clinical guidelines recommended by the U.S. Preventive Services Task Force.
  - Recommend a referral if these criteria apply:
    o Ashkenazi Jewish heritage
    o History of ovarian cancer at any age in the patient or any first- or second-degree relatives
    o Any first-degree relative with a history of breast cancer diagnosed before the age of 50 years
    o Two or more first- or second-degree relatives with a breast cancer diagnosis at any age
    o Relative with a diagnosis of bilateral breast cancer (or the patient)
    o History of breast cancer in a male relative

PSYCHOSOCIAL HEALTH AND FUNCTIONING

- Body image

  - Most patients have dealt with body image issues prior to the survivorship period.
  - Patients may have deferred reconstruction but now feel they are "well" enough to discuss this topic. Or they may be dissatisfied with the cosmetic effects of the current reconstruction. Referral to plastic surgery is indicated.
  - Obesity may be a problem. Attempt to motivate survivors into a comprehensive weight loss program that includes dietary and exercise counseling if indicated.
  - If patients still feel uncomfortable with their bodies, refer to a psychologist or sexuality program.
  - Ask patients about their sexuality and activity with their partner. If they express problems with orgasm, relationship concerns, or intimacy, refer for sexuality counseling. Rule out painful intercourse and address the problem (refer to monitoring for late effects).

- Relationship issues

  - Inquire about family status, peer relationships, and community and social involvement. Refer to social services as indicated.

- Access to primary care specialists

  - Assess interdisciplinary health providers. It is essential to have a primary care provider and cardiologist if indicated. An endocrinologist may be needed to discuss adequate bone health care. Psychology/psychiatry may be indicated for depression; refer to social services.

- Financial issues

  - Financial stress resulting from the treatment phase of care and ongoing life changes may be substantial.
    o Refer to social services as indicated.
    o Provide lists of available community and national organizations.

CLINICAL VIGNETTE

PM, a 59-year-old woman who developed invasive ductal carcinoma of the left breast 6 years ago, has transitioned to survivorship care. Her cancer was estrogen receptor–positive/progesterone receptor–positive and human epidermal growth factor receptor-2 negative. She received neoadjuvant paclitaxel followed by a regimen of fluorouracil, doxorubicin, and cyclophosphamide. She underwent segmental mastectomy and axillary lymph node dissection followed by radiation to the left breast. She completed 5 years of anastrozole therapy and is now receiving extended therapy. PM's mother had breast cancer at age 70, and a cousin had colon cancer at age 63.

1. Posttreatment, this patient should be closely monitored for
   A. Bone mineral density
   B. Endometrial cancer
   C. Peripheral neuropathy
   D. A and C only
   E. All of the above

2. As part of her survivorship care, laboratory studies should include
   A. Complete blood count (CBC) and liver function tests
   B. Carcinoembryonic antigen (CEA) and tumor markers CA 15-3 or CA 27.29
   C. Vitamin D level
   D. A and B only
   E. All of the above

3. This patient is at risk for
   A. Angiosarcoma within the radiation field
   B. Breast cancer
   C. Thyroid cancer

    D. A and B only

    E. All of the above

4. PM arrives at your clinic as a new patient. You should pay particular attention to

    A. Her body mass index

    B. The date of her last Pap smear

    C. The date of her last colonoscopy

    D. B and C only

    E. All of the above

5. A serious potential late effect of this patient's treatment is

    A. Cardiac valve dysfunction

    B. Kidney function impairment

    C. Congestive heart failure

    D. Pulmonary function impairment

    E. Menopausal symptoms

Answers

1. D

Bone density loss is a concern related to this patient's age and menopausal status and is an untoward effect from taking anastrozole. Chemotherapy-induced peripheral neuropathy (CIPN) is a common treatment-related adverse effect from chemotherapy agents including paclitaxel, which can affect long-term quality of life. Paclitaxel peripheral neuropathy improves for most patients during the months after cessation of treatment, but it may persist and pose a long-term problem. CIPN typically occurs in a symmetric, distal, "glove and stocking" distribution. The neuropathy predominantly consists of sensory, rather than motor, symptoms. Anastrozole, unlike tamoxifen, does not act on the uterine lining and does not increase risk for endometrial cancer.

2. C

Vitamin D levels are important to monitor as part of osteoporosis screening and bone health surveillance. Based on existing evidence, routine laboratory tests including CBC, liver function tests, CEA, and tumor markers (CA 15-3 or CA 27.29) are not recommended for otherwise asymptomatic patients with no specific findings upon clinical examination.

3. D

When compared with the general population, breast cancer survivors are at slightly higher risk for developing a second cancer within the first 10 years after a first diagnosis. Breast cancer survivors are at elevated risk for a second primary breast cancer, especially women with a family history of breast cancer. Second cancers can be attributed to common risk factors that predisposed to the first cancer (e.g., genetic risk, environmental risk) or to treatment-related effects. PM's family history does not suggest a hereditary cancer syndrome. Survivors who had radiation are at a slightly higher risk for angiosarcoma in the treatment field, which typically appears as a purple or nodular lesion and necessitates biopsy.

4. E

Risk reduction and early detection is an important domain of survivorship care. In the absence of symptoms or clinical findings, PM should follow routine screening recommendations for her age and risk status for cervical and colorectal cancers. Obesity is associated with increased risk for contralateral breast, endometrial, and colorectal secondary primary cancers.

5. C

The cardiotoxic effects of anthracycline can produce irreversible cardiomyopathy that can progress to late-onset heart failure. Patients may be asymptomatic initially, and ventricular dysfunction, heart failure, and arrhythmias may occur later, even decades after the discontinuation of anthracycline therapy. The cardiotoxic effects are dose dependent, and a careful history that takes into account the cumulative dose of doxorubicin will assist in risk assessment. PM should be monitored for symptoms that suggest heart failure. If applicable, manage hypertension and encourage smoking cessation, weight loss, and physical activity to help reduce cardiac risk. Cardiac valve, renal function, and pulmonary function decline are not anticipated late effects of chemotherapy or radiation to the breast. Menopausal symptoms, whether the result of natural aging or premature ovarian failure, are common and bothersome but rarely serious.

RECOMMENDED READINGS

American Cancer Society. *Breast Cancer Facts & Figures 2015–2016.* Atlanta, GA: American Cancer Society; 2015.

American College of Obstetricians and Gynecologists, Committee on Gynecologic Practice. *The Use of Vaginal Estrogen in Women With a History of Estrogen Dependent Breast Cancer.* Committee Opinion 659. Available at: https://www.acog.org/-/media/Committee-Opinions/Committee-on-Gynecologic-Practice/co659.pdf?dmc=1&ts=20170925T1259379102. Published March 2016.

American Congress of Obstetricians and Gynecologists Committee on Practice B-G. ACOG Practice Bulletin No. 126: management of gynecologic issues in women with breast cancer. *Obstet Gynecol.* 2012;119(3):666–682. doi:10.1097/AOG.0b013e31824e12ce

Chung KC, Kim HJ, Jeffers LL. Lymphangiosarcoma (Stewart–Treves syndrome) in postmastectomy patients. *J Hand Surg Am.* 2000;25(6):1163–1168. doi:10.1053/jhsu.2000.18490

Cozen W, Bernstein L, Wang F, et al. The risk of angiosarcoma following primary breast cancer. *Br J Cancer*. 1999;81(3):532–536. doi:10.1038/sj.bjc.6690726

Druesne-Pecollo N, Touvier M, Barrandon E, et al. Excess body weight and second primary cancer risk after breast cancer: a systematic review and meta-analysis of prospective studies. *Breast Cancer Res Treat*. 2012;135(3):647–654. doi:10.1007/s10549-012-2187-1

Howell A, Cuzick J, Baum M, et al. Results of the ATAC (Arimidex, Tamoxifen, Alone or in Combination) trial after completion of 5 years' adjuvant treatment for breast cancer. *Lancet*. 2005;365(9453):60–62. doi:10.1016/S0140-6736(04)17666-6

Howlader N, Noone AM, Krapcho M, et al. SEER Cancer Statistics Review, 1975–2013, based on November 2015 SEER data submission. Available at: http://seer.cancer.gov/csr/1975_2014. Published April 2016.

Kaplan HG, Malmgren JA, Atwood MK. Increased incidence of myelodysplastic syndrome and acute myeloid leukemia following breast cancer treatment with radiation alone or combined with chemotherapy: a registry cohort analysis 1990–2005. *BMC Cancer*. 2011;11:260. doi:10.1186/1471-2407-11-260

Khatcheressian JL, Hurley P, Bantug E, et al. Breast cancer follow-up and management after primary treatment: American Society of Clinical Oncology clinical practice guideline update. *J Clin Oncol*. 2013;31(7):961–965. doi:10.1200/JCO.2012.45.9859

Levi F, Randimbison L, Te VC, La Vecchia C. Increased risk of esophageal cancer after breast cancer. *Ann Oncol*. 2005;16(11):1829–1831. doi:10.1093/annonc/mdi363

Miller KD, Siegel RL, Lin CC, et al. Cancer treatment and survivorship statistics, 2016. *CA Cancer J Clin*. 2016;66(4):271–289. doi:10.3322/caac.21349

Molina-Montes E, Requena M, Sánchez-Cantalejo E, et al. Risk of second cancers cancer after a first primary breast cancer: a systematic review and meta-analysis. *Gynecol Oncol*. 2015;136(1):158–171. doi:10.1016/j.ygyno.2014.10.029

Narod SA, Iqbal J, Giannakeas V, et al. Breast cancer mortality after a diagnosis of ductal carcinoma in situ. *JAMA Oncol*. 2015;1(7):888–896. doi:10.1001/jamaoncol.2015.2510

Neugut AI, Lee WC, Murray T, et al. Lung cancer after radiation therapy for breast cancer. *Cancer*. 1993;71(10):3054–3057. doi:10.1002/1097-0142(19930515)71:10<3054::AID-CNCR2820711027>3.0.CO;2-N

Schmitz K. Physical activity in breast cancer survivors. In: Courneya KSF, Christine M, eds. *Physical Activity and Cancer*. New York, NY: Springer; 2011.

Willer A. Reduction of the individual cancer risk by physical exercise. *Onkologie*. 2003;26(3):283–289. doi:10.1159/000071626

Yap J, Chuba PJ, Thomas R, et al. Sarcoma as a second malignancy after treatment for breast cancer. *Int J Radiat Oncol Biol Phys*. 2002;52(5):1231–1237. doi:10.1016/S0360-3016(01)02799-7

11   Colorectal Cancer Survivorship Care

George J. Chang
Tilu Ninan

CLINICAL PEARLS

If a patient's carcinoembryonic antigen (CEA) level has been elevated in the past, CEA should be checked two to four times yearly for the first 3 years and then once or twice annually.

- Adjuvant chemotherapy may be associated with long-term toxicities, including myelosuppression, peripheral neuropathy, memory loss, and cognitive decline.

- Following curative treatment, patients should undergo annual surveillance computed tomography (CT) scans of the chest, abdomen, and pelvis for 5 years.

- Many survivors (particularly following rectal cancer treatment) experience bowel dysfunction that may involve an increase in bowel movement frequency, irregularity, incomplete evacuation, clustering, incontinence, urgency or inability to defer defecation, and loss of sensation or discrimination. These events can affect a survivor's activities of daily living and social activities. Treatment should be individualized to a patient's particular symptoms.

- Survivorship care following colorectal cancer treatment should emphasize management of psychosocial concerns, treatment-associated toxicity, and health promotion in addition to recurrence detection.

COLORECTAL CANCER EPIDEMIOLOGY AND SURVIVORSHIP CARE

- Colorectal cancer background:
  - Third most common cancer in both men and women
  - Second leading cause of death in men and women combined
  - Colorectal cancer deaths have been declining because of improvements in early detection and treatment

- Incidence of colorectal cancer in the general population is declining because of increased screening
- Premalignant lesions (polyps) and early-stage disease may not produce symptoms; therefore, screening is important to identify and remove polyps before they become cancerous.
- Colorectal cancer most often affects people ages 50 and older, but incidence is rising in the younger population. Screening is recommended for average-risk individuals beginning at age 45 to 50.
- Risk for colorectal cancer increases as people get older.
- A personal or family history of colorectal cancer or adenomatous polyps, inherited genetic mutations, and inflammatory bowel disease may increase risk for colorectal cancer.
- Incidence of colorectal cancer is higher in developed countries than in developing countries.
- Colorectal cancer incidence is highest among Black people; Asian and Pacific Islanders have the lowest incidence of colorectal cancer.
- Colorectal cancer incidence is slightly higher for men.

- Overview of colorectal cancer types:

  - Colon and rectal cancer:
    - Incidence:
      — Between 2004 and 2013, the incidence of colorectal cancer declined by 3% per year in adults 50 years of age and older.
      — During the same period, incidence of colorectal cancer in patients younger than age 50 has increased by 2% per year, with a larger increase in rectal versus colon cancers.
      — Among colorectal cancers, 95% are adenocarcinomas.
      — A genetic syndrome is the cause of approximately 5% of colorectal cancers.
      — Lynch syndrome (hereditary nonpolyposis colorectal cancer) is the most common genetic syndrome associated with colorectal cancer. This syndrome also increases risk for endometrial and ovarian cancers and several other cancers. It typically is associated with an earlier age at onset than sporadic colorectal cancer.
      — Familial adenomatous polyposis (FAP) is the second most common genetic syndrome associated with colorectal cancer. Patients with FAP also are at risk for duodenal cancer, desmoid tumors, thyroid cancer, and several other cancers and other conditions. FAP is associated with hundreds to thousands of polyps and early age at colorectal cancer onset. Common treatment includes prophylactic colectomy.
      — MUTYH-associated polyposis and hamartomatous polyposis conditions (Peutz–Jeghers syndrome, juvenile polyposis syndrome, and Cowden syndrome) also are associated with colorectal cancers.

    o Mortality:
       — Between 2005 and 2014, the mortality rate associated with colorectal cancer declined by 2.5% per year, but colorectal cancer remains a major cause of cancer-related death, affecting an estimated 49,190 people in 2016 and representing 8.3% of all cancer deaths.
    o Survival rate:
       — Survival rates are dependent upon stage at diagnosis.
       — The 5-year overall survival rate for colorectal cancer is approximately 65%, whereas the 10-year survival rate is 58%. However, survival is higher than 90% when cancers are detected early.
       — For patients with localized disease, the 5-year relative survival rate is 90.1%.
       — For patients with regional-stage disease, the 5-year relative survival rate is 71.2%.
       — For patients with distant-stage disease, the 5-year relative survival rate is 13.5%.

- Clinical tools to guide care of colorectal cancer survivors:

  - Eligibility criteria for transition of patients with colon cancer to survivorship care (refer to Figure 11.1)
  - Eligibility criteria for transition of patients with rectal cancer to survivorship care (refer to Figure 11.2)

- Disease surveillance:

  - Medical history and physical examination:
    - Obtain a complete history and perform a general examination.
    - Ask the survivor about symptoms such as fatigue, change in appetite, pain, and unexplained weight loss; these symptoms may be signs of cancer recurrence or metastatic disease.
    - Ask about respiratory symptoms and perform lung auscultation. The lung is a common site for metastasis, especially for patients with a history of rectal cancer.
    - Ask about any abdominal symptoms, especially bowel pattern changes, abdominal pain, nausea, vomiting, blood in the stool, black stool, and rectal bleeding, which can signal local recurrence or metachronous primary tumors.
    - Perform an abdominal examination. Palpate for any masses in the abdomen or hepatomegaly—colorectal cancer can metastasize to the peritoneum and liver.
    - Assess the stoma if one is present. Note the color and any bleeding or discharge from the stoma. Ask about ostomy output.
    - Assess for genitourinary symptoms; colorectal cancer (particularly rectal cancer) recurrence or treatment can cause urinary and sexual dysfunction.
    - Ask about bone pain to assess for metastatic disease to bone. Ask about pain in the lower back, pelvis, hip, groin, or buttocks to assess for pelvic insufficiency

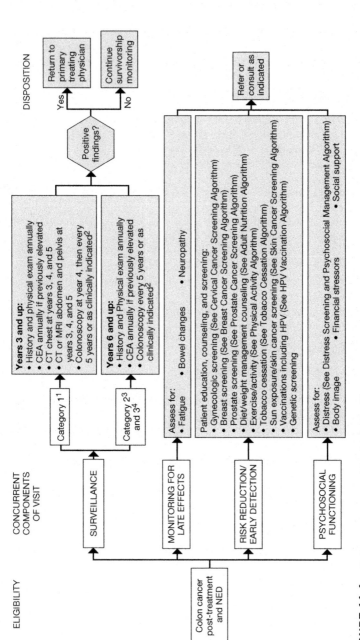

FIGURE 11.1 Colon cancer survivorship algorithm.

NED, no evidence of disease; [1]Category 1: Stage I, no evidence of disease at 3 years; [2]Colonoscopic surveillance is recommended at 1 year following resection, then (if normal) after 3 more years, then (if normal) once every 5 years; [3]Category 2: Stages II and IIIA–B, no evidence of disease at 5 years; [4]Category 3: Stages IIIC and IV, no evidence of disease at 5 years. *Source:* Copyright 2016 The University of Texas MD Anderson Cancer Center.

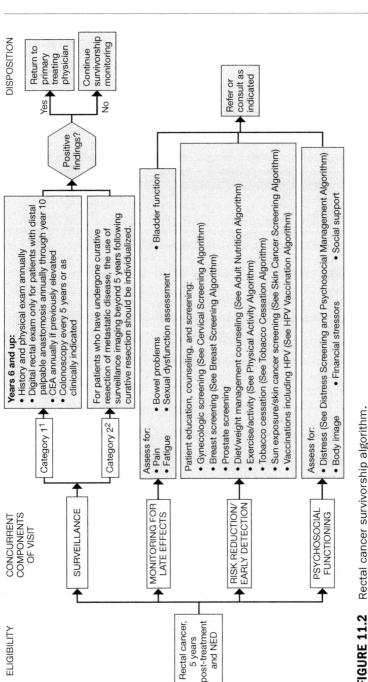

FIGURE 11.2 Rectal cancer survivorship algorithm.

Note: Clinical risk is based on preoperative staging (clinical stage) vs. pathologic staging, which is based on the postoperative tumor specimen (for patients who were unable to receive neoadjuvant therapy); NED, no evidence of disease; [1]Category 1: Localized, Stages I–III; [2]Category 2: Metastatic, Stage IV. *Source:* Copyright 2016 The University of Texas MD Anderson Cancer Center.

fracture, particularly for patients who undergo pelvic radiation therapy as part of their cancer treatment.

o Ask about any swelling or mass in the groin, neck, or axilla to evaluate for lymphadenopathy.

o Ask about neurological symptoms including memory or behavior changes, unbalanced walking, headache, dizziness, seizures, speech or vision changes, weakness, or numbness and tingling to assess for metastatic disease in the brain or peripheral neuropathy associated with treatment.

o An annual digital rectal examination should be performed for rectal cancer survivors with distal palpable anastomosis.

■ Order diagnostic testing based on examination findings or a patient's symptoms.
■ Diagnostic testing:

o Laboratory tests:

— If a patient's CEA level has been elevated in the past, CEA should be checked two to four times yearly for the first 3 years and then annually.

— Other laboratory testing should be based on a patient's symptoms or examination findings.

o Radiologic procedures:

— Chest CT to evaluate for possible metastasis to the lungs

a. Annually for 5 years (stages II–III)

— CT or MRI of the abdomen and pelvis to evaluate for intra-abdominal or locoregional recurrence

b. Annually for 5 years (stages II–III)

— Other diagnostic testing should be ordered based on a patient's symptoms or examination findings

— There is no need for routine PET examinations

o Special procedures:

— Colonoscopy to assess for local recurrence and for new primary colorectal cancer or polyps

a. At year 1 after initial surgical treatment

b. Subsequent examinations every 3 to 5 years depending upon findings

MONITORING FOR LATE EFFECTS

• Adjuvant chemotherapy may be associated with long-term toxicities including myelosuppression, peripheral neuropathy, memory loss, and cognitive decline. Primary management includes supportive care and referral for specialty care as needed:

■ Patients who received adjuvant chemotherapy with oxaliplatin may experience long-term effects of peripheral neuropathy with cold and hot intolerance and loss of sensation or proprioception, which can impact balance. These patients' symptoms may need to be managed supportively, or referral to a neurologist can be initiated:

o Oxaliplatin treatment is associated with portal hypertension with hypersplenism; thrombocytopenia; and perisplenic, perigastric, or peristomal varices.

Portal hypertension may be associated with variceal bleeding and should be suspected in patients who have thrombocytopenia or varices identified upon radiographic or physical examination.

- Many survivors (particularly following rectal cancer treatment) experience bowel dysfunction that may involve an increase in nighttime bowel movements, irregularity, incomplete evacuation, clustering, incontinence, urgency or inability to defer defecation, and loss of sensation or discrimination. These events can affect a survivor's activities of daily living and social activities. Treatment should be individualized to a patient's particular symptoms:

  - Obtain a careful history to gain a complete understanding of bowel habits to make the appropriate recommendations. Exacerbation of bowel frequency and clustering often indicates incomplete evacuation; avoid the temptation to administer antidiarrheal medication. Incomplete evacuation can be treated with bulk-forming agents or intermittent laxatives to induce more complete emptying (e.g., a patient may report a cyclical pattern of several days of "good" bowel function with few bowel movements, during which time the colon is filling with incompletely evacuated stool, followed by 1 to 2 days of markedly increased bowel movements signaling the evacuation phase).
  - Proactively manage bowel function with strategies that include laxative-induced evacuation followed by antidiarrheal-induced decreased motility to prevent urgent bowel movements.
  - Incontinence should be managed with perianal care strategies to avoid perianal irritation and pain. Some patients may benefit from daily enema therapy to facilitate evacuation and avoid daytime incontinence.
  - Patients with ostomies also may have ostomy-related concerns including parastomal hernia or poor appliance fitting. Consultation with wound ostomy and continence nursing specialists or a colorectal surgeon may be helpful.

- Pelvic radiation therapy is associated with bowel, bladder, sexual, and gonadal dysfunction and can increase risk for pelvic insufficiency fractures or other pelvic malignancies. Symptoms that suggest fractures should be evaluated. Primary management is supportive, including pain management and promotion of bone health. Radiation also can cause ovarian failure and induce premature menopause in women; men will experience infertility. Primary management is supportive.

- Urogenital dysfunction is seen in colorectal cancer survivors as a result of surgery and radiation therapy. Assess for urinary symptoms of either incomplete emptying with urinary retention or decreased bladder capacity with urinary urgency.

- Symptoms of sexual dysfunction such as dyspareunia, vaginal dryness, erectile dysfunction, and ejaculation problems should be assessed and treated accordingly. If needed, refer to urology or gynecology. Vaginal stenosis also can contribute to dyspareunia after pelvic radiation. These patients should be referred to gynecology.

- Refer to Chapter 3 for more information about treatment-related late and long-term effects.

RISK REDUCTION AND EARLY DETECTION

- Cancer screening:

  ▪ Refer to Chapter 5 for general cancer screening recommendations. Colorectal cancer survivors should follow cancer screening guidelines for other cancers.
  ▪ Colon cancer screening with colonoscopy should be performed every 5 years or sooner depending upon findings at the previous colonoscopy or the need for symptom evaluation.
  ▪ People with a history of colorectal cancer are at increased risk for a second colorectal cancer. This risk is even higher if a patient had his or her first diagnosis before age 50:
    o History of adenomatous polyps increases risk for colorectal cancer.
    o Adenomatous colon polyps can become cancerous if they are not removed. Colonoscopy allows for identification and removal of these polyps to stop progression to colon cancer.
    o Patients with colon cancers associated with genetic mutations (e.g., Lynch syndrome or FAP) should be referred to appropriate specialists for screening for associated cancers. Refer to screening guidelines for endometrial cancer and ovarian cancers for patients with Lynch syndrome.

- Dietary changes may help reduce colorectal cancer risk. Encourage patients to maintain a healthy diet:

  ▪ Advise patients to avoid excess consumption of processed meats.
  ▪ Encourage daily consumption of fruits and vegetables.
  ▪ Promote a high-fiber diet.
  ▪ Consumption of whole grain instead of refined grain products may protect against colorectal cancer.

- Exercise:

  ▪ People who engage in regular exercise are at lower risk for colorectal cancer.

- A higher risk for colorectal cancer death is associated with patients who do not lead an active lifestyle.

  ▪ The American Cancer Society recommends 150 minutes of moderate-intensity activity or 75 minutes of vigorous activity per week.

- Encourage a healthy body weight:

- Obesity is strongly associated with an increased risk for a variety of cancers including colorectal cancer and young age at onset.
- Obesity also is associated with an increased risk for colorectal cancer recurrence.
- Aspirin:
  - Aspirin is associated with reduced risk for developing colorectal cancer or death from colorectal cancer.
- Alcohol:
  - Consumption of moderate to heavy alcohol (three or more drinks per day) is associated with increased risk for colorectal cancer.
  - The American Cancer Society recommends no more than one alcoholic drink per day for women and no more than two alcoholic drinks per day for men.
- Tobacco:
  - There is an association between colorectal cancer and death from colorectal cancer and tobacco smoking.
  - Smokers should be counseled about the risks associated with tobacco use, and tobacco cessation assistance should be offered.

PSYCHOSOCIAL HEALTH AND FUNCTIONING

- Distress:
  - Refer to MD Anderson's clinical practice algorithm, Distress Screening and Psychosocial Management of Adult Cancer Patients (available at www.mdanderson.org).
  - Anxiety and fear of recurrence are among the primary concerns for patients with colorectal cancer. These patients may not have a clear understanding of recurrence causes and their underlying risks. Education on recurrence risks over time may help to alleviate anxiety.
  - Colorectal cancer survivors may experience long-term treatment-related toxicities that affect their activities of daily living and result in impaired quality of life or depression. Ask survivors if they are experiencing these symptoms
  - Sexual dysfunction also can contribute to distress. Refer to sexuality counseling as needed.
- Relationship issues:
  - A survivor's relationships with family and friends may be affected by treatment and long-term effects of treatment.
  - Ask survivors about support they receive from family and friends and the communication between them.
  - Provide information about support groups.
  - Refer to social services as needed.

- Body image issues:

  - Physical changes following treatment, including the presence of an ostomy, can affect body image for colorectal cancer survivors. Ask survivors to discuss their thoughts about these issues.
  - Provide education about ostomy care and diet to help alleviate anxieties about odor, flatulence, and so forth.
  - Incontinence or fear of incontinence may also cause body image issues. Ask about incontinence issues and educate regarding effective management.
  - Refer to social services, wound ostomy continence nursing specialists, support groups, or psychology/psychiatry services as needed.

- Financial distress:

  - The financial burden associated with treatment can cause substantial distress and have a dramatic impact on a patient and his or her family's financial stability. Furthermore, the physical and psychosocial burdens associated with cancer treatment can decrease a patient's likelihood of returning to work:
    o One in three patients will experience financial distress.
    o Long-term effects of cancer treatment such as neuropathy, fatigue, and bowel and bladder pattern changes may affect a survivor's ability to continue performing their job tasks. Help patients assess their employment-related status and navigate job changes as needed.
    o For survivors with ostomy and incontinence issues, bear in mind that costs associated with necessary medical supplies may cause financial stress.
    o Severe financial distress among patients with cancer is associated with increased mortality and overall poorer well-being, impaired health-related quality of life, and diminished quality of care.
    o Refer to a social worker and/or case manager as needed.
    o Provide information about support groups that may be helpful with these issues.
    o Help patients complete Family and Medical Leave Act forms if needed.

CLINICAL VIGNETTE

RRL is a 74-year-old male who was diagnosed with rectal cancer 6 years ago. He received neoadjuvant chemoradiation therapy, which consisted of external beam radiation and concurrent capecitabine. RRL's next treatment included a low anterior resection and temporary ileostomy, which has since been reversed and subsequent adjuvant chemotherapy with 5-FU and oxaliplatin.

Questions

1. Posttreatment, this patient should be closely monitored for
   A. Sexual dysfunction
   B. Urinary dysfunction
   C. Peripheral neuropathy

D. All the above

E. Only A and C

2. The most serious immediate posttreatment malignancy risk for this patient is
   A. Prostate cancer
   B. Skin cancers
   C. Liver cancer
   D. All of the above
   E. None of the above

3. RRL arrives at your clinic as a new patient. You should pay particular attention to his
   A. Bowel history
   B. Healthcare associated stress and anxiety
   C. Diet, weight, and level of exercise
   D. All of the above
   E. Only A and B

4. A significant potential late treatment effect that is particularly concerning when considering this patient's age and treatment is
   A. Sexual dysfunction
   B. Chronic flatus
   C. Pelvic insufficiency fracture
   D. Undiagnosed diabetes
   E. Unresolved fatigue

Answers

1. D

Following chemoradiation and surgery for rectal cancer, patients are at risk for bowel dysfunction that includes urgency, frequency, incomplete evacuation with clustering, and incontinence. Symptoms vary among patients as not all patients will experience symptoms or have the same severity of symptoms. These symptoms are often driven by incomplete evacuation resulting in intermittent episodes of fecal frequency. These symptoms are also known as low anterior syndrome and are characterized by a validated symptom scale. Generally, patients at this stage in their survivorship continuum will experience little further change in their bowel function as most changes (improvement) occur during the first 24 months after surgery. Management options include bulk-forming agents (e.g., supplemental fiber) and antimotility and promotility agents. Patients with refractory symptoms may be considered for colostomy.

Autonomic dysfunction including bowel, bladder, and sexual dysfunction can occur following pelvic surgery and are exacerbated by pelvic radiotherapy. Causes of dysfunction include direct injury to nerves during surgery or radiation and ongoing nerve injury due to surrounding fibrosis. Body image concerns should also be addressed not only in patients with permanent ostomies but also in patients experiencing significant bowel dysfunction. Body image issues can also lead to sexual dysfunction. Treatment with oxaliplatin is frequently associated with peripheral neuropathy and long-lasted effects are observed in at least 10% of patients. Therefore, this patient should be monitored for symptoms of peripheral neuropathy.

2. A

The risks and benefits of prostate cancer screening should be discussed with the patient so that he can make an informed decision about prostate cancer screening. Given the patient's age and sex, he should be considered for age appropriate prostate cancer screening. The history of rectal cancer is not specifically associated with an increased risk for any of the cancers listed; however, all patients should undergo risk assessment (e.g., history of sun exposure, chronic hepatitis, etc.) for all potential cancers and should be appropriately referred. Given that, the patient is 6 years following treatment of his rectal cancer and his risk for developing metastasis is very low; however, unexplained symptoms suggestive of tumor recurrence should be worked up.

3. D

In this patient following low anterior resection, the bowel history should be assessed. The patient should be asked about his bowel habits including frequency, difficulty with defecation or need for straining, stool caliber, completeness of evacuation, incontinence, or other issues that indicate an anatomic problem (e.g., stricture) or debilitating low anterior resection syndrome. In addition, the patient should be assessed for hematochezia or alteration in bowel habits that could suggest local tumor recurrence or a new primary cancer. Indeed, it should be confirmed that the patient is up to date on their screening colonoscopies. Because bowel, bladder, and sexual dysfunction can be complications of rectal cancer treatment, associated symptoms should be assessed. Treatment related bowel, bladder, and sexual dysfunction can lead to problems with body image and depression.

Some patients may also experience financial stressors with severe anxiety because of the costs associated with treatment, and these stressors may be long lasting. Some patients may still experience a significant degree of anxiety associated with fear of recurrence that is persistent despite the long duration following treatment and associated reduction in recurrence risk. Patient should be asked about these and appropriate referral should be initiated as needed.

Finally, all patients should be encouraged to maintain a healthy diet, healthy weight, and exercise regularly. Healthy behaviors are associated with lower risk for cancer recurrence, lower risk for development of new cancers, improved emotional well-being, and in this population, improved bowel function.

4. C

Pelvic insufficiency fractures can be a potential late treatment effect of radiation therapy to the pelvis. It can be associated with debilitating pain and is a particular problem in postmenopausal women. The patient should be assessed for symptoms of pelvic fracture. Although this patient is also at risk for treatment-related sexual dysfunction or an alteration in flatus, including increase, these concerns generally manifest early in the posttreatment period; however, insufficiency fractures are a late effect.

RECOMMENDED READINGS

Ahmed SU, Eng C. Colorectal cancer survivorship management. In: Foxhall LE, Rodriguez MA, eds. *Advances in Cancer Survivorship Management*. New York, NY: Springer Publishing; 2015:71–93. doi:10.1007/978-1-4939-2986-5

American Cancer Society. Colorectal Cancer Facts and Figures 2014-2016. Atlanta, GA: 2014:428–455. doi:10.3322/caac.21286

American Cancer Society. Cancer Facts and Figures 2017. Atlanta, GA: 2017.

Anderson AS, Steele R, Coyle J. Lifestyle issues for colorectal cancer survivors—perceived needs, beliefs and opportunities. *Support Care Cancer*. 2013;21(1):35–42. doi:10.1007/s00520-012-1487-7

Berian J, Cuddy A, Francescatti AB, et al. A systematic review of patient perspectives on surveillance after colorectal cancer treatment. *J Cancer Surviv*. 2017;11:542–552. doi:10.1007/s11764-017-0623-2

Cao Y, Nishihara R, Wu K, et al. Population-wide impact of long-term use of aspirin and the risk for cancer. *JAMA Oncol*. 2016;2(6):762–769. doi:10.1001/jamaoncol.2015.6396

Chen TY, Emmertsen KJ, Laurberg S. Bowel dysfunction after rectal cancer treatment: a study comparing the specialist's versus patient's perspective. *BMJ Open*. 2014;4(1):e003374. doi:10.1136/bmjopen-2013-003374

Chu KM. *Epidemiology and Risk Factors of Colorectal Cancer*. Philadelphia, PA: Saunders; 2011:doi:10.1016/B978-1-4160-4686-8.50006-3

Denlinger CS, Barsevick AM. The challenges of colorectal cancer survivorship. *J Natl Compr Canc Netw*. 2009;7(8):883–893; quiz 894. doi:10.6004/jnccn.2009.0058

Desch CE, Benson AB 3rd, Somerfield MR, et al. Colorectal cancer surveillance: 2005 update of an American Society of Clinical Oncology practice guideline. *J Clin Oncol*. 2005;23(33):8512–8519. doi:10.1200/JCO.2005.04.0063

Earle CC, Ganz PA. Cancer survivorship care: don't let the perfect be the enemy of the good. *J Clin Oncol*. 2012;30(30):3764–3768. doi:10.1200/JCO.2012.41.7667

El-Shami K, Oeffinger KC, Erb NL, et al. American Cancer Society colorectal cancer survivorship care guidelines. *CA Cancer J Clin*. 2015;65(6):428–455. doi:10.3322/caac.21286

Faul LA, Shibata D, Townsend I, Jacobsen PB. Improving survivorship care for patients with colorectal cancer. *Cancer Control.* 2010;17(1):35–43. doi:10.1177/107327481001700105

Giardiello FM. *Hereditary Colorectal Cancer and Polyp Syndromes.* Philadelphia, PA: Saunders; 2011:21–30. doi:10.1016/B978-1-4160-4686-8.50006-3

Huxley RR, Ansary-Moghaddam A, Clifton P, et al. The impact of dietary and lifestyle risk factors on risk of colorectal cancer: a quantitative overview of the epidemiological evidence. *Int J Cancer.* 2009;125(1):171–180. doi:10.1002/ijc.24343

Jasperson KW, Tuohy TM, Neklason DW, et al. Hereditary and familial colon cancer. *Gastroenterology.* 2010;138(6):2044–2058. doi:10.1053/j.gastro.2010.01.054

National Cancer Institute Surveillance, Epidemiology, and End Results Program. Cancer stat facts: colon and rectum cancer. Available at https://seer.cancer.gov/statfacts/html/colorect.html

Siegel RL, Miller KD, Jemal A. Cancer statistics, 2016. *CA Cancer J Clin.* 2016;66(1):7–30. doi:10.3322/caac.21332

Steele SR, Chang GJ, Hendren S, et al. Practice guideline for the surveillance of patients after curative treatment of colon and rectal cancer. *Dis Colon Rectum.* 2015;58(8):713–725. doi:10.1097/DCR.0000000000000410

Zafar SY. Financial toxicity of cancer care: it's time to intervene. *J Natl Cancer Inst.* 2016;108(5):1–4. doi:10.1093/jnci/djv370

12

Prostate Cancer Survivorship Care

Jeri Kim
Spyridon Basourakos
William Osai

CLINICAL PEARLS

- Consider monitoring lipid metabolism parameters (total cholesterol, tri-glycerides, low-density lipoprotein, and high-density lipoprotein) in all men treated with androgen deprivation therapy (ADT).

- Patients may request a penile prosthesis to treat erectile dysfunction (ED). Patients with these devices should be monitored for pain and skin changes that may indicate malfunction.

- Men treated with ADT and some who received radiation therapy are at elevated risk for osteopenia, osteoporosis, and bone fracture because of loss in bone mineral density. A bone mineral density test is recommended to monitor bone health.

PROSTATE CANCER EPIDEMIOLOGY

- General background:

  - The prostate is a gland in the male reproductive system that is located in front of the rectum, below the bladder, and behind the base of the penis.
  - The prostate is responsible for the production of most semen.
  - Approximately one in seven men will be diagnosed with prostate cancer during their lifetime.
  - The average age at prostate cancer diagnosis is 66 years, and almost 60% of prostate cancer cases are diagnosed in men older than age 60.
  - African American men and men with a family history of prostate cancer are at increased risk.

- ▪ Prostate cancer is the second most common cause of cancer death in men and the most common nonskin cancer in men.
- ▪ Survival rates are better when prostate cancer is diagnosed at an early stage and disease is localized.
- ▪ Histologic types of prostate cancer:
  - o Adenocarcinoma (almost all cases)
  - o Small-cell carcinomas
  - o Neuroendocrine tumors
  - o Transitional-cell carcinomas
  - o Sarcomas

- Overview: Prostate cancer stages:

  - ▪ Localized prostate cancer:
    - o Disease has not spread outside of the gland.
    - o Almost 90% of newly diagnosed prostate cancer cases.
    - o Clinical symptoms are rare, and most cases are detected through elevated prostate-specific antigen (PSA) levels.
  - ▪ Advanced prostate cancer:
    - o Disease is extended outside of the gland and involves surrounding structures or has metastasized to distant sites.
    - o Patients commonly have symptoms of the lower urinary tract such as blood in urine, need for frequent urination, or pain during urination.
    - o Five-year survival for locally advanced and metastatic prostate cancer is nearly 30%.

- Adenocarcinoma: The most prevalent prostate cancer type:

  - ▪ Incidence:
    - o Second most common cancer among American men
    - o Accounts for approximately 200,000 new cases in the United States annually
    - o Incidence increases with age
  - ▪ Mortality: Most men with prostate cancer die of other causes, and many never know they have it.
  - ▪ Survival:
    - o The 5-, 10-, and 15-year relative survival rates are 99%, 98%, and 95%, respectively, when all prostate cancer stages are included.

- Clinical tools to guide care for prostate cancer survivors:

  - ▪ Eligibility criteria for transition to survivorship care:
    - o Patients should be at 2 or more years beyond treatment completion and have no evidence of recurrence (refer to Figure 12.1).

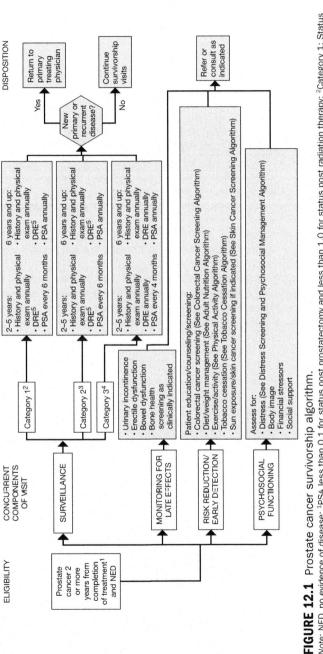

FIGURE 12.1 Prostate cancer survivorship algorithm.

Note: NED, no evidence of disease; [1]PSA less than 0.1 for status post prostatectomy and less than 1.0 for status post radiation therapy; [2]Category 1: Status post radical prostatectomy or radiation therapy: Pathologic stage pT2, N0, M0, negative margins, or clinical stage cT2, N0, M0, Gleason less than or equal to 7 and PSA less than 0.1 ng/mL or less than 1 ng/mL if treated with radiation therapy; [3]Category 2: Status post prostatectomy or status post prostatectomy plus radiation therapy, pathologic stage >T2, N0, M0, positive margins, Gleason less than or equal to 7, PSA less than 0.1 ng/mL; [4]Category 3: Status post prostatectomy or status post prostatectomy plus radiation therapy or status post radiation therapy: Pathologic staging pT3, N0, M0, clinical stage cT3, N0, M0, Gleason 8–10, and PSA less than 0.1 ng/mL or less than 1 ng/mL if treated with radiation therapy only; [5]DRE, digital rectal examination as clinically indicated if PSA is undetectable. *Source:* Copyright 2016 The University of Texas MD Anderson Cancer Center.

DISEASE SURVEILLANCE

- Medical history and examination:

  - General examination:
    - o Risk for prostate cancer recurrence is dependent on Gleason grade, surgical stage, clinical cancer stage, and surgical margin status. Recurrence occurs usually within 2 years after primary treatment ends; however, recurrence can occur at any time after primary treatment. A detectable PSA level after surgery or a rising PSA level after radiation therapy is the first sign of recurrence, but symptomatic recurrences also are possible when PSA levels are undetectable.
    - o Ask the patient about systemic symptoms such as weight loss, night sweats, fatigue, and focal bone pain.
    - o Review the patient's vital signs, blood pressure, body mass index, and pulse.

  - Head and neck examination:
    - o Examine the head, hair, scalp, and neck areas. If focal pain is noted in the scalp, bony face, or neck, obtain an x-ray of the area.
    - o Neck: Perform systematic palpation of the nodal chains of the head and assess the neck and range of motion of the cervical spine. If lymph nodes are enlarged in the head and neck area, a biopsy is recommended. Restricted range of motion or pain with range of motion should warrant CT or x-ray.
    - o Palpate the thyroid for nodules/masses. A sonogram is needed to characterize a nodular thyroid. If biopsy is indicated, refer to an endocrinologist.
    - o Eye examination: Although rare, eye metastasis from prostate cancer has been reported. Funduscopic examination is recommended. Visual acuity changes should be assessed by an ophthalmologist.

  - Thoracic examination:
    - o Examine the supraclavicular, infraclavicular, and axillary lymph nodes for enlargement. Enlarged nodes should be considered for biopsy.
    - o Ribs: Palpate the ribs and thoracic spine to assess for pain. If the patient reports focal pain, x-ray is recommended. A bone scan may be needed if bone pain is present at other sites.
    - o Lungs: Auscultate all lung fields. Ask about new-onset or worsening wheezing, shortness of breath, cough, or hemoptysis. Recommend chest x-ray and refer to a pulmonologist for mediastinal adenopathy, pleural effusion, or lung infiltrates.
    - o Breast: Examine breasts for gynecomastia and tenderness. Most survivors should not have persistent gynecomastia far into the survivorship period. Refer to endocrinology for persistent gynecomastia.

  - Cardiovascular examination:
    - o Auscultate heart sounds. Note rate, rhythm, and murmur presence, especially in patients who received ADT who are at higher risk for cardiovascular disease (myocardial infarction, coronary atherosclerosis, and sudden cardiac death and stroke).

- Examine the pulse and cardiac rhythm for irregularities. Note the point of maximum impulse. An electrocardiogram is recommended to assess new rhythms. New-onset shortness of breath or activity intolerance warrants an echocardiogram or cardiologist referral.
    - Auscultate for carotid bruits. A cardiology referral and carotid ultrasound are recommended if a carotid bruit is noted.
    - Examine for pedal edema, which may be an early sign of heart failure, especially in men treated with ADT.
    - Observe for lower extremity lymphedema in men who underwent pelvic lymph node dissection.
- Abdominal examination:
    - Gastrointestinal (GI) manifestation as a first sign of prostate cancer recurrence is rare but has been reported. Men who received radiation therapy are more likely to report GI symptoms.
    - Ask patients who have received radiation therapy about new-onset nausea, vomiting, decreased appetite, hematemesis, abdominal discomfort, weight loss, rectal bleeding, or worsening constipation or diarrhea.
    - Observe the abdomen for hernias (men who have had a prostatectomy). Men with an enlarging hernia may need surgery.
    - Auscultate for bowel sounds. An abdominal x-ray may be needed when slow bowel sounds suggest constipation (particularly for patients who received radiation therapy). Increased fiber intake is the recommended treatment for constipation.
    - Palpate the liver and spleen. Perform superficial and deep palpation of all abdominal quadrants to assess for masses or tenderness:
      — New-onset abdominal tenderness or masses should be evaluated with a CT scan as needed. Colonoscopy is recommended for new-onset GI bleeding, especially for patients who receive radiation therapy.
- Genitourinary examination:
    - Ask patients about urinary and bowel incontinence. Note characteristics of urinary incontinence (Figure 12.1, Table 12.1). Ask about quality of erectile function (Figure 12.1, Table 12.1). Ask about the presence of a new penis curvature or plaque (for patients using intracavernosal injections and those who have had radical prostatectomy).
    - Palpate the entire length of the penis for plaque (hardening of tissue):
      — Pertinent to men on intracavernosal injections
    - Examine the anus for hemorrhoids or fissures (especially for patients who receive radiation therapy)
    - Digital rectal examination:
      — Palpate for symmetry, size, and nodularity in men treated with radiation therapy.
      — Palpate for abnormal growth in the prostatic fossa in men treated with radical prostatectomy.
    - Urinary frequency, urgency, intermittency, and retention warrant urologist referral.
    - Unsatisfactory erectile ability warrants referral to an ED specialist.

- Musculoskeletal examination:
  - o Systemic musculoskeletal effects are uncommon among prostate cancer survivors; however, ADT exposure may affect muscle mass.
  - o Examine muscle tone and body fat composition if a change in body composition is suspected.
  - o Evaluate muscle strength in the upper and lower extremities.
  - o Ask about new-onset focal bony pain:
    — In the setting of protracted bone pain, x-ray is recommended to assess for sclerotic bone lesions. Lytic bone lesions are rare.
  - o Examine the lower extremities for edema:
    — Patients may develop venous obstruction in the pelvis after lymph node dissection or radiation.
    — Unilateral or worsening edema should be worked-up with venous Doppler to rule out deep vein thrombosis.
    — Patients with lymphedema should be referred for specialized physical therapy.
- Neurologic examination:
  - o Evaluate cranial nerves for abnormalities:
    — Visual changes warrant brain magnetic resonance imaging or CT.
    — New-onset neck pain or submental pain should warrant CT of the head and neck and a whole-body bone scan to rule out skull base and submental metastasis.
  - o Palpate the entire spine for focal tenderness or pain:
    — Patients with upper or lower extremity sensory or motor function changes should undergo imaging of the spine to rule out vertebral metastasis impinging on the spinal cord.
    — Patients with suspected spinal cord involvement should be referred for multidisciplinary care with a radiation oncologist and neurosurgeon.
- Mental health examination:
  - o Assess mentation:
    — Patients with cognitive dysfunction should be sent for a psychometric evaluation.
  - o Assess psychosocial status:
    — Ask about sexual function and coping and ask both the patient and his significant other if ED is an issue. Recommend a consultation with a sexual therapist.
    — Advise patients who are distressed by urinary incontinence about available treatment options. Psychological counseling is indicated if quality of life is affected.

- Laboratory tests:

  - Check total serum PSA level at every visit. Ultrasensitive PSA is not recommended. An undetectable PSA level for patients who underwent prostatectomy and stable PSA levels lower than 2 ng/mL are the targets.
  - Order a complete blood count with differential if anemia is suspected.

- Order a lipid profile (to monitor high-density lipoprotein [HDL] and triglycerides) and fasting blood glucose to assess for metabolic syndrome in men treated with ADT.
- Order a bone mineral density test, testosterone, and vitamin D levels in men treated with ADT to monitor bone health. Refer to an endocrinologist if osteopenia or osteoporosis is evident.
- Radiologic testing:
- Bone mineral density, bone scan, and bone x-ray are screening modalities:
  o Assess for systemic disease.
  o Monitor bone health.
- CT scan:
  o Assess lymph nodes and viscera as dictated by symptoms.

Monitoring for Late Effects

- Cardiovascular risk and symptom assessment:

  - Patients who received ADT with or without antiandrogen are at higher risk for diabetes, sarcopenia, coronary artery disease, myocardial infarction, and sudden cardiac death even in the absence of prior heart disease, and risk remains after ADT is discontinued. Consider monitoring lipid metabolism parameters (total cholesterol, triglycerides, low-density lipoprotein, and HDL) in all men treated with ADT.
  - Men who receive ADT should be screened for diabetes and begin treatment if necessary. When present, hypertension should be treated to prevent coronary disease progression.
  - Obesity and sarcopenia are more likely in men who received ADT; these men experience changes in body composition attributable to increased body fat mass and decreased lean muscle mass. Patients should be encouraged to engage in physical activity and follow a plant-based diet.

- Urinary dysfunction:

  - Urinary dysfunction (urinary frequency, urgency, weak stream, hesitancy, and retention) are common among patients with prostate cancer after treatment. Patients who undergo prostatectomy regain maximum control at about 1 year and stabilize. Patients who received radiation therapy experience incontinence gradually and stabilize after about 1 to 2 years. Patients who receive radiation therapy may experience hematuria. Validated instruments such as the American Urological Association Symptom Index should be used to regularly assess patient status. Consult urology regarding worsening symptoms (Table 12.1).

- ED:

  - Prostate cancer survivors develop ED regardless of therapy received. Those who undergo prostatectomy experience more severe ED but recover maximally by 2 years. Patients who have radiation therapy experience a less dramatic decline in erectile function. Oral phosphodiesterase-5 inhibitors such as Cialis, Viagra,

TABLE 12.1 Potential Late Effects of Prostate Cancer Therapy: Screening and Interventions

Late Effect	Screening Tool	Recommended Intervention
ED	IIEF[a] or EPIC-CP[b]	Refer to an ED specialist for persistent issues
Urinary incontinence	AUA[c]	Refer to a urologist for worsening lower urinary tract symptoms
Anxiety/depression/fear of cancer recurrence		Refer for psychotherapy or psychiatric care; use pharmacotherapy as needed
Gastrointestinal symptoms (constipation and/or diarrhea)	Screen for colorectal cancer using American Cancer Society guidelines[d]	If screening colonoscopy findings are negative, pharmacotherapy for constipation and diarrhea and dietary modification (increase fiber)
Second cancers (for patients who receive radiation therapy)	Colorectal cancer screening using ACS guidelines[d]	Follow American Cancer Society guidelines
Bone health (for men who received androgen deprivation therapy)	Bone mineral density test (dual-energy x-ray absorptiometry scan)	Refer to National Osteoporosis Foundation[e] guidelines
Cardiovascular and metabolic effects	Assess weight, blood pressure, and lipid and blood glucose levels	Follow national guidelines from the United States Protective Services Task Force[f] and the American Heart Association[g]

[a]International Index of Erectile Function: This index assesses male sexual function domains of erectile function, orgasmic function, sexual desire, intercourse satisfaction, and overall satisfaction.

[b] Expanded Prostate Cancer Index Composite for Clinical Practice: This clinical tool monitors urinary, bowel, sexual, and vitality/hormonal health.

[c]American Urologic Association Symptom Index: This index consists of seven questions covering frequency, nocturia, weak urine stream, hesitancy intermittence, incomplete emptying, and urgency.

[d]American Cancer Society Guidelines for Screening and Early Detection of Colon Cancer.

[e]National Osteoporosis Foundation Guidelines for Osteoporosis Prevention, Detection, and Treatment.

[f]United States Protective Services Task Force Recommendations for Screening for Cardiovascular Risk Factors.

[g]American Heart Association Guidelines for Screening for Cardiovascular Risks.

and Levitra offer relief. Recommend ED specialist care if these medications are ineffective. Erectile function should be assessed with validated tools such as the International Index of Erectile Function (IIEF) (Table 12.1).

■ Patients may request a penile prosthesis to treat ED. Patients with these devices should be monitored for pain and skin changes that may indicate malfunction.

■ Patients who receive ADT may never recover normal testosterone levels. If a low androgen level is implicated in ED, consult with a urologist about supplementation. Testosterone replacement is not recommended for patients who undergo radiation therapy.

- Bowel function:

  ■ Men treated with radiation therapy are at elevated risk for constipation, diarrhea, or incontinence. Recommend colonoscopy for patients with new-onset bowel function changes. Recommend increased fiber intake to avoid constipation or antidiarrheal medications to avoid uncomplicated loose stools.

- Bone health:

  ■ Men treated with ADT and some who received radiation therapy are at elevated risk for osteopenia, osteoporosis, and bone fracture because of bone mineral density loss. A bone mineral density test is recommended to monitor bone health. Follow National Osteoporosis Foundation guidelines when treating these patients (Table 12.1).

  ■ Physical activity and weight-bearing exercises are recommended.

- Infertility:

  ■ Younger men with prostate cancer lose the ability to ejaculate after treatment. Recommend fertility preservation before treatment.

  ■ Refer to a fertility specialist if a man who wants children did not use a sperm bank prior to receiving treatment.

RISK REDUCTION/EARLY DETECTION FOR SURVIVORS

- Refer to Chapter 5 to review guidelines on cancer screening and human papilloma virus (HPV) vaccinations.

- Correlation between prostate cancer survivors and secondary malignancies:

  ■ Prostate cancer survivors treated with radiation therapy are at a small increased risk for secondary cancers of the bladder and colon.

  ■ Patients who report new-onset hematuria should be referred to a urologist for a complete evaluation to rule out bladder cancer.

  ■ Patients who report new-onset melena or hematochezia or a change in bowel habits should be referred for a colonoscopy to rule out colon cancer.

- Vaccinations:

  - A yearly influenza vaccination is recommended unless a patient is allergic to the vaccine. Pneumococcal and shingles vaccinations also are recommended. The shingles vaccination is not recommended in patients who are immunocompromised.

- Frequently refer to the American Society of Clinical Oncology Survivorship Guidelines (frequently updated online) and American Cancer Society recommendations (also frequently updated online).

PSYCHOSOCIAL HEALTH AND FUNCTIONING

- Distress:

  - Refer to MD Anderson's clinical practice algorithm, Distress Screening and Psychosocial Management of Adult Cancer Patients (available at www.mdanderson.org).
  - Prostate cancer survivors are at risk for general distress, anxiety, and major depressive disorders related to fear of disease recurrence, ED, and incontinence. Use Health-Related Quality of Life tools to assess patients who exhibit mood changes.
  - Involve family and partners in the evaluation of patient mental and social health; some patients do not report their full extent of distress. For example, African Americans with cancer may be less likely to seek psychosocial services.

- Relationship issues:

  - Some prostate cancer survivors do not recover erectile function after treatment, stay incontinent of urine, and develop bowel control symptoms that can affect body image and intimate relationships.
  - Inquire about family status and social and professional activities during encounters.
  - Spouses and partners should be involved in the management of known treatment effects. Promote open communication and refer for sexual counseling as needed.
  - Assess single, divorced, or widowed survivors for support needs. Single men are more likely to need support.
  - Refer to support groups, counselors, and peers for support.

- Financial issues:

  - Out-of-pocket expenses for cancer survivors continue after active treatment ends. Copay, insurance deductible, and prescription and nonprescription medication and supply costs can be a burden for low-income young and fixed-income older survivors:
    o Assess the survivor's ability to meet expenses.
    o Help survivors access the most convenient and least costly survivorship care.
    o Link qualified survivors to Medicaid and Social Security.
  - Refer to a social worker or case manager

CLINICAL VIGNETTE

Harold is a 66-year-old African American prostate cancer survivor. After several years of monitoring his PSA level, he was diagnosed with prostate cancer. When his PSA level reached 5.3 ng/mm, he underwent a transrectal ultrasound-guided prostate biopsy that yielded 12 cores. Seven cores revealed prostate adenocarcinoma with a Gleason score of 7 (3 + 4) in three cores and score of 6 (3 + 3) in four cores. He was treated with robot-assisted radical prostatectomy (bilateral nerve sparing) and limited pelvic lymph node dissection. Final surgical pathology revealed a Gleason score of 7 (3 + 4) in both lobes but without extraprostatic extension. Twelve pelvic lymph nodes (six from each side) were negative for metastatic disease. His PSA level was undetectable for 1 year following surgery, but it rose from 0.2 ng/mL to 0.8 ng/mL over the next year and he was referred for salvage radiation therapy. After confirming that he had no metastatic disease, he received 70 Gy of external beam radiation therapy plus 6 months of ADT, after which his PSA level became undetectable. Harold has decided to move his care to your clinic instead of seeing an oncologist. He comes in for his annual visit.

Questions

1. According to the prostate cancer staging classification, Harold's cancer stage should be classified as
   A. Localized prostate cancer
   B. Advanced prostate cancer
   C. Metastatic prostate cancer
   D. None of the above

2. Based on this patient's medical history, which condition could be a late therapy effect?
   A. ED
   B. Urinary incontinence and/or retention
   C. Hematuria
   D. All of the above

3. ADT treatment poses risk for
   A. Cardiovascular disease
   B. Osteopenia and/or loss of muscle mass
   C. Dyslipidemia
   D. All of the above

4. Which blood tests are appropriate for this patient?
   A. PSA level only
   B. PSA and testosterone levels only
   C. PSA and lipid levels only
   D. PSA, testosterone, and lipid levels

Answers

1. A
According to the American Joint Committee on Cancer Guidelines and prostate cancer staging principles, prostate cancer confined within the prostate is considered localized. Prostate cancer that has spread beyond the prostate capsule but is confined to the pelvis is locally advanced, and prostate cancer that has spread beyond the pelvis is metastatic.

2. D
Prostate cancer treatment involving radiation therapy, radical prostatectomy, or both with or without ADT can cause any of these conditions. Local treatment affects the neurovascular and the muscular structures and can result in urethral stricture, severing of the neurovascular bundles involved in erection, and inflammation of the bladder mucosa. Patients who have urinary incontinence or retention should be referred to a urologist for evaluation. ED should be managed with oral phosphodiesterase five inhibitors. Surgical implantation of a penile prosthesis is an option for motivated and appropriate patients.

3. D
ADT, even when administered for only 6 months, is associated with increased risk for cardiovascular disease and dyslipidemia. Long-term ADT is associated with osteopenia, osteoporosis, and changes in body fat and muscle composition. Prostate cancer survivors who are exposed to ADT should be screened for dyslipidemia, tested for osteopenia/osteoporosis, and encouraged to engage in resistance exercise to regain and maintain muscle mass.

4. D
Because Harold was treated with radical prostatectomy, radiation therapy, and ADT, only PSA and lipid level bloodwork are needed. The total serum PSA level should be undetectable in the setting of prostate gland excision. Testosterone levels must be monitored after ADT exposure. Serum testosterone level will recover in most men, indicating the effects of ADT are not lingering; however, when testosterone remains at castrate level, close monitoring for adverse effects is warranted. Castration-level testosterone correlates with increased risk for cardiovascular morbidity, so continued monitoring of lipid metabolism parameters and treatment as indicated is recommended.

RECOMMENDED READINGS

Albadainah F, Khader J, Salah S, et al. Choroidal metastasis secondary to prostatic adenocarcinoma: case report and review of literature. *Hematol Oncol Stem Cell Ther.* 2015;8(1):34-37.

Barry MJ, Fowler FJ Jr., O'Leary MP, et al. The American Urological Association Symptom Index for Benign Prostatic Hyperplasia. *J Urol.* 2017;197(2 Suppl):S189-S197.

Bienz M, Saad F. Androgen-deprivation therapy and bone loss in prostate cancer patients: a clinical review. *Bonekey Rep.* 2015;4:716.

Cosman F, de Beur SJ, LeBoff MS, et al. Clinician's guide to prevention and treatment of osteoporosis. *Osteoporos Int.* 2014;25(10):2359-2381.

Elabbady A, Kotb AF. Unusual presentations of prostate cancer: a review and case reports. *Arab J Urol.* 2013;11(1):48-53.

Fuentes-Raspall R, Inoriza JM, Rosello-Serrano A, et al. Late rectal and bladder toxicity following radiation therapy for prostate cancer: predictive factors and treatment results. *Rep Pract Oncol Radiother.* 2013;18(5):298-303.

Goff DC Jr., Lloyd-Jones DM, Bennett G, et al. 2013 ACC/AHA Guideline on the Assessment of Cardiovascular Risk: a report of the American College of Cardiology/ American Heart Association Task Force on Practice Guidelines. *J Am Coll Cardiol.* 2014;63(25 Pt B):2935-2959.

Hong MK, Kong J, Namdarian B, et al. Paraneoplastic syndromes in prostate cancer. *Nat Rev Urol.* 2010;7(12):681-692.

Levin B, Levin TR, Lieberman DA, et al. screening and surveillance for the early detection of colorectal cancer and adenomatous polyps, 2008: a joint guideline from the American Cancer Society, the US Multi-Society Task Force on colorectal cancer, and the American College of Radiology. *Gastroenterology.* 2008;134(5):1570-1595.

Lin JS, Piper MA, Perdue LA, et al. Screening for colorectal cancer: updated evidence report and systematic review for the US Preventive Services Task Force. *JAMA.* 2016;315(23):2576-2594.

Maines F, Caffo O, Veccia A, Galligioni E. Gastrointestinal metastases from prostate cancer: a review of the literature. *Future Oncol.* 2015;11(4):691-702.

Margel D, Baniel J, Wasserberg N, et al. Radiation therapy for prostate cancer increases the risk of subsequent rectal cancer. *Ann Surg.* 2011;254(6):947-950.

Morgia G, Russo GI, Tubaro A, et al. Prevalence of cardiovascular disease and osteoporosis during androgen deprivation therapy prescription discordant to EAU guidelines: results from a multicenter, cross-sectional analysis from the CHOsIng Treatment for Prostate canCEr (CHOICE) Study. *Urology.* 2016;96:165-170.

Nguyen PL, Alibhai SM, Basaria S, et al. Adverse effects of androgen deprivation therapy and strategies to mitigate them. *Eur Urol.* 2015;67(5):825-836.

Nieder AM, Porter MP, Soloway MS. Radiation therapy for prostate cancer increases subsequent risk of bladder and rectal cancer: a population based cohort study. *J Urol.* 2008;180(5):2005-2010.

Petrakis D, Pentheroudakis G, Kamina S, et al. An unusual presentation of a patient with advanced prostate cancer, massive ascites and peritoneal metastasis: case report and literature review. *J Adv Res.* 2015;6(3):517-521.

Qaseem A, Snow V, Shekelle P, et al. Screening for osteoporosis in men: a clinical practice guideline from the American College of Physicians. *Ann Intern Med.* 2008;148(9):680-684.

Rosen RC, Riley A, Wagner G, et al. The international index of erectile function (IIEF): a multidimensional scale for assessment of erectile dysfunction. *Urology.* 1997;49(6):822-830.

Siegel RL, Miller KD, Jemal A. Cancer statistics, 2017. *CA Cancer J Clin.* 2017;67(1):7-30.

Skolarus TA, Wolf AM, Erb NL, et al. American Cancer Society Prostate Cancer Survivorship Care Guidelines. *CA Cancer J Clin.* 2014;64(4):225-249.

Smith RA, Andrews K, Brooks D, et al. Cancer screening in the United States, 2016: a review of current American Cancer Society guidelines and current issues in cancer screening. *CA Cancer J Clin.* 2016;66(2):96-114.

Stephenson AJ, Scardino PT, Kattan MW, et al. Predicting the outcome of salvage radiation therapy for recurrent prostate cancer after radical prostatectomy. *J Clin Oncol.* 2007;25(15):2035-2041.

Suardi N, Porter CR, Reuther AM, et al. A nomogram predicting long-term biochemical recurrence after radical prostatectomy. *Cancer.* 2008;112(6):1254-1263.

Vodermaier A, Linden W, Siu C. Screening for emotional distress in cancer patients: a systematic review of assessment instruments. *J Natl Cancer Inst.* 2009;101(21): 1464-1488.

Walker LM, Wassersug RJ, Robinson JW. Psychosocial perspectives on sexual recovery after prostate cancer treatment. *Nat Rev Urol.* 2015;12(3):167-176.

Wallis CJ, Mahar AL, Choo R, et al. Second malignancies after radiotherapy for prostate cancer: systematic review and meta-analysis. *BMJ.* 2016;352:i851.

Zelefsky MJ, Levin EJ, Hunt M, et al. Incidence of late rectal and urinary toxicities after three-dimensional conformal radiotherapy and intensity-modulated radiotherapy for localized prostate cancer. *Int J Radiat Oncol Biol Phys.* 2008;70(4):1124-1129.

Zheng Z, Yabroff KR, Guy GP Jr, et al. Annual medical expenditure and productivity loss among colorectal, female breast, and prostate cancer survivors in the United States. *J Natl Cancer Inst.* 2016;108(5).

Zumsteg ZS, Spratt DE, Romesser PB, et al. Anatomical patterns of recurrence following biochemical relapse in the dose escalation era of external beam radiotherapy for prostate cancer. *J Urol.* 2015;194(6):1624-1630.

Head and Neck Cancer Survivorship Care

Kristen B. Pytynia
Charles Schreiner IV

CLINICAL PEARLS

- Ask survivors about any changes in breathing, voice quality, eating (including difficulty swallowing and coughing/choking when eating different consistencies), pain in the head and neck (especially ear), and head and neck masses.
- Head and neck cancer survivors may experience some degree of swallowing dysfunction ranging from prolonged eating time to a complete inability to orally ingest nutrition or hydration.
- Dysphagia can lead to slow and/or noisy eating, causing embarrassment, and social isolation.

EPIDEMIOLOGY OF HEAD AND NECK CANCERS

- Head and neck cancers affect the soft tissues of the head and neck. Cancer type and anatomical origin determine treatment choice:

- Salivary cancers:
  - o The salivary glands consists of two paired parotid glands, two paired submandibular glands, two paired sublingual glands, and thousands of small minor salivary glands distributed throughout the oral cavity.
  - o Cancer can arise from any component of the salivary gland, and there are more than 30 types of salivary gland cancers. The most common types are adenoid cystic carcinoma, mucoepidermoid carcinoma, and lymphoma.
  - o The parotid and submandibular glands are the most common locations for salivary cancers.
  - o The mainstay of treatment for salivary gland carcinoma (not lymphoma) is surgery, often followed by postsurgical radiation.
  - o Adenoid cystic carcinoma in particular has a propensity to travel on nerves and can cause late recurrences in nerve tissue as well as neuropathy.
  - o Salivary gland cancer is relatively unusual, accounting for less than 1% of all cancer cases.
  - o The facial nerve is embedded within the parotid gland, and parotid cancer or surgery may affect facial nerve function.

■ Squamous cell cancers:
  o Larynx/hypopharynx:
    — The larynx is composed of the glottis, or true vocal cords; the supraglottis (epiglottis and everything above the true vocal cords); and the subglottis. Tumors most commonly arise in the glottis and supraglottis. Glottic tumors will cause early symptoms of hoarseness. Supraglottic tumors often are not detected until they have spread to the lymph nodes.
    — Patients also may experience referred pain to the ear. Hypopharyngeal cancers most commonly arise in the piriform sinuses (the mucosa next to the voice box).
    — Tobacco use causes laryngeal and hypopharyngeal tumors. The incidence of these cancers decreases as tobacco use decreases.
    — In 2015, nearly 14,000 cases of laryngeal cancer were diagnosed in the United States.
    — Chemotherapy and radiation are used in the setting of advanced tumors in an attempt to preserve the larynx; this technique is known as *organ preservation*.
    — Surgical treatment to address advance tumors of the larynx and hypopharynx is total laryngectomy:
      a. Patients who undergo total laryngectomy have a stoma in the neck and are permanent neck breathers.
      b. They can be intubated only through a neck stoma, not through the mouth.
  o Oral cavity:
    — Squamous cell carcinoma in the oral cavity most commonly arises from the lateral tongue.
    — Tobacco and alcohol use are risk factors, but this cancer also can occur in nonsmokers.
    — In 2013, 30,000 people in the United States received an oral cancer diagnosis. Oral cavity cancer is the most common cancer in India because of betel nut use (a type of chewing tobacco).
    — Primary treatment for any oral cavity cancer is surgery. Advanced lesions may necessitate reconstruction and postsurgical radiation.
  o Oropharynx:
    — Oropharyngeal squamous cell cancer can occur in the tissue at the base of the tongue, tonsils, or the walls of the pharynx.
    — There is an epidemic increase in the incidence of oropharyngeal cancer. These increases are caused by the human papilloma virus (HPV).
    — Between 2008 and 2012, approximately 15,000 people received an oropharyngeal cancer diagnosis each year, 12,500 of whom were men.
    — By the end of 2019, there will likely be more men with HPV-related oropharyngeal cancer than women with HPV-related cervical cancer.
    — There is no screening modality for oropharyngeal cancer.

— The HPV vaccine series can protect future generations against HPV-related cancers.

— Men in their forties and fifties with no smoking history are most likely to develop HPV-related oropharyngeal cancer.

— Patients often present with enlarged neck lymph nodes that they notice while shaving.

— Primary treatment is radiation with or without chemotherapy, although some trials describe use of transoral robotic surgery.

o Nasopharynx:

— Nasopharyngeal squamous cell carcinoma usually arises from the fossa of Rosenmüller, which is the tissue adjacent to the eustachian tube.

— Patients often present with adenopathy and nasal obstruction or cranial neuropathy:

— Nasopharyngeal cancer is endemic in China and thought to be related to the Epstein–Barr virus and other environmental and genetic factors. It is less common in the United States.

Disease Surveillance

• Medical history and physical examination:

■ General examination:

o The physical examination must focus on the head and neck.

o Ask the survivor about any changes in breathing, voice quality, eating (including difficulty swallowing and coughing/choking when eating different consistencies), pain in head and neck (especially ear), and head and neck masses.

■ Review the patient's vital signs.

• Head and neck examination:

■ Providers may use any headlight that allows for use of both hands to retract tissue and view all pertinent areas:

o Skin and soft tissues of the head and neck:

— Assess for trauma, lesions, or other abnormalities such as facial asymmetry and facial motor weakness.

— Any obvious masses or growths should warrant further evaluation.

— Lymphedema commonly occurs after radiation treatment and can be symptomatic. A specialized physical therapist can teach the patient daily massage techniques.

o Ears:

— It is important to evaluate the external auditory canal in patients with a history of radiation treatment for nasopharynx, sinus, and cutaneous cancers:

a. If an impacted cerumen is encountered, this should be removed under binocular microscopy.

b. Assess for exposed bone in the ear canal.

— A middle ear evaluation via the appearance of the tympanic membrane is important, especially for patients who describe aural fullness, ear pain, and/ or decreased hearing

    a. The presence of an effusion, either serous or purulent, should lead the provider to perform a fiberoptic nasopharyngoscopy to assess for a nasopharyngeal mass causing Eustachian tube dysfunction. Radiation scarring may be another cause.

o Eyes:

— Fundus examination: Risk for accelerated development of cataracts is associated with orbital irradiation. If patients are symptomatic (experiencing a change in vision or glare at night), they should be referred to an ophthalmologist for a complete eye examination.

o Nasal cavity: A nasal speculum helps practitioners visualize the nasal cavity and the sinus turbinates:

— Assess for evidence of sinus drainage, mucosal edema, and/or epistaxis.

— The nasal cavity can be extremely dry after radiation therapy.

— Antiangiogenic systemic therapy can also cause mucosal dryness.

o Oral cavity:

— Assess for ulcers, leukoplakia, visible masses, or mucosal changes.

— Assess the patient's dental health and hygiene, looking for evidence of dental decay or oral dryness.

— Be sure to evaluate the floor of the mouth and the hard and soft palates.

— Pay particular attention to the lateral tongue as a potential recurrence site.

o Oropharynx: A mirror examination (indirect laryngoscopy) is a good noninvasive method with which to evaluate the inferior oropharyngeal structures, although performing the examination can be a challenge depending on patient tolerance:

— The tonsils, if present, should be inspected for any obvious asymmetry or neoplasia.

— The base of the tongue, viewed via an indirect mirror or a fiberoptic scope examination, should be evaluated for asymmetry, mucosal ulceration, mucosal bleeding, and/or friability.

o Larynx/hypopharynx:

— Fiberoptic laryngoscopy:

    a. Laryngoscopy is an excellent tool with which to monitor patients with laryngeal or hypopharyngeal cancer who have been treated with organ preservation (radiation with or without chemotherapy).

    b. Ask the patient to stick out his or her tongue; this generally allows for base-of-tongue visualization.

    c. Ask the patient to puff out his or her cheeks; this may help the provider to adequately visualize the hypopharyngeal structures, including the piriform sinuses.

— A mirror examination (indirect laryngoscopy) also may be helpful.

— Refer to an otolaryngologist to address concerning findings.

- Palpation:
  - Palpate the entire oral cavity and oropharynx with a gloved hand:
    — The floor of mouth, oral tongue, buccal mucosa, hard and soft palates, tonsils (or tonsillar pillars), and the base of the tongue need to be palpated and assessed for masses, nodules, asymmetric fullness, and friability.

    — If a mucosal lesion is present, it is likely causing pain, so the palpation examination should be performed quickly and not repeated unless necessary.

    — If a mass or lump is detected in the floor of the mouth, the provider can place one hand under the patient's chin and attempt to bimanually isolate the lump to perform a detailed palpable examination.
  - Examine lymphatic nodes in preauricular, submental, submandibular, postauricular, occipital, and cervical (both superficial and deep) neck areas; if any node is larger than 1.5 cm, fine needle aspiration (FNA) biopsy is recommended.
  - Thyroid palpation for nodules/masses: If palpable nodules/masses are suspected, a thyroid ultrasound is recommended; FNA or palpable mass biopsy may be indicated based on ultrasound results.
- Auscultation:
  - For patients who received neck external beam radiation therapy, the bilateral carotid arteries should be auscultated to assess for bruits. In the event of a positive finding, the patient should be referred to a cardiologist/vascular specialist.
  - This is especially important for patients who have experienced stroke-like symptoms or have difficulty controlling their blood pressure.

- Laboratory tests:

  - Order thyroid function studies (thyroid-stimulating hormone and T4) annually or more often if a patient is experiencing new symptoms or has had neck irradiation:
  - If a patient is a melanoma survivor, check his or her lactate dehydrogenase level annually.
  - If performing a CT scan with contrast enhancement, check renal function (with blood urea nitrogen and creatinine labs) prior to contrast administration.

- Radiologic procedures:

  - A chest x-ray must be performed at least annually to monitor for changes in parenchyma or nodal areas or signs of aspiration pneumonia (Figure 13.1):
    - Chest x-ray findings will reveal if a patient is experiencing aspiration and/or developing lung cancer (metastatic or new primary) or mediastinal adenopathy.
    - Positive findings should be followed-up with a chest CT.
    - Patients who have received previous neck irradiation will likely have some scarring of the lung apices.

158

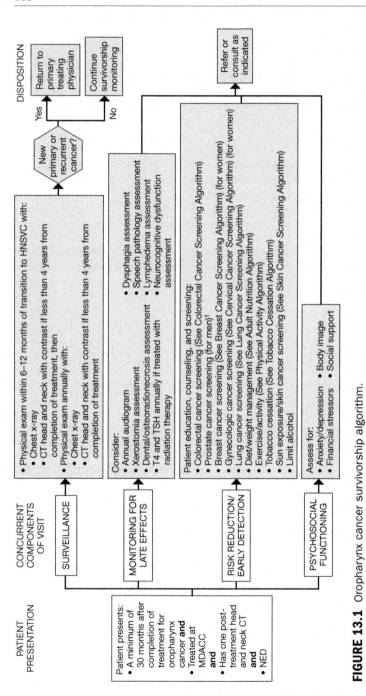

FIGURE 13.1 Oropharynx cancer survivorship algorithm.

NED, no evidence of disease; HNSVC = Head and Neck Survivorship clinic; [1]Based on American Cancer Society Prostate Cancer Screening Guidelines.

Source: Copyright 2017 The University of Texas MD Anderson Cancer Center.

- Cross-sectional imaging (CT and MRI) may be used to monitor lesions that are not amenable to direct inspection (salivary gland, nasopharynx, hypopharynx). There is controversy regarding whether cross-sectional imaging should be included in screening.
- PET scans should not be used for screening because of the high rate of false positives. PET scans are useful only when a known tumor is present.
- Ultrasound of the neck soft tissues is useful when evaluating:
  o Oral tongue cancer survivors
  o Cutaneous cancer survivors
  o Thyroid cancer survivors

Monitoring for Late Effects

- Lung function and cancer screening:

  - Patients who are active smokers or those who have had lung radiation exposure from mediastinal or upper body nodal radiation are at risk for secondary primary lung cancers. Smoking cessation is strongly urged for active smokers.

- Orbital examination:

  - Cataract risk is associated with orbital irradiation:
    o Survivors of nasopharyngeal, paranasal sinus, and some oropharyngeal cancers are at elevated risk for late effects if they received radiation therapy because of proximity to the lens.
  - Eye dryness also may develop and can be exacerbated if a patient has diabetes. Artificial tears are recommended.
  - These patients should be referred to an ophthalmologist for a yearly complete eye examination.

- Hearing loss:

  - Platinum-based chemotherapies including cisplatin and carboplatin are used in the systemic treatment of many head and neck cancers:
    o This class of medication may be given in concert with other chemotherapeutic agents, concurrently with radiation therapy, and sometimes both.
    o Hearing loss is a known side effect of this class of chemotherapy; in particular, cisplatin may result in permanent hearing loss.
  - Radiation to the acoustic nerve and/or the cochlear system may also result in hearing loss.
  - An annual audiogram and referral to an audiologist may be considered if a survivor experiences hearing changes:
    o A baseline audiogram is recommended if a patient was treated with platinum-based chemotherapy.

- Oral cavity late effects:

  - Patients with a previous head and neck cancer and a smoking history are at elevated risk for secondary malignancies. Squamous cell carcinoma can develop on any mucosal surface.

  - Oral dryness also may occur, although newer radiation techniques substantially decrease this side effect. Patients need to drink water frequently to moisten their mouth, and artificial saliva may be helpful.

  - There may be accelerated dental decay:
    o Fluoride gel prophylaxis is recommended.
    o Patients need dental cleanings on a frequent and regular basis and should be monitored by their dentist.
    o Patients who have had radiation to the head and neck region should not have dental extractions unless cleared by a dental oncologist. Radiation can cause osteoradionecrosis in which bone is infected, exposed, and often painful. This problem can be severe.

- Dysphagia:

  - Dysphagia can occur as a result of surgery or radiation and may be progressive even years after treatment.

  - Swallowing exercises and compensatory methods may improve swallowing, and patients should be followed by a speech pathologist.

  - Severe dysphagia may result in aspiration. Repeated aspiration can be fatal.

- Endocrine system evaluation:

  - Thyroid examination:
    o Patients may develop hypothyroidism if they have received radiation to the upper thorax/mediastinum or the head and neck region.
    o This may occur soon after therapy or many years later.

  - Thyroid function monitoring is recommended throughout a patient's lifespan:
    o This should be done at least annually and sooner if a patient experiences new-onset or worsening fatigue, facial edema (myxedema), or weight gain.

- Cranial neuropathy:

  - New-onset cranial neuropathy (facial nerve, trigeminal nerve) can be a sign of recurrent cancer or late effects of radiation (glossopharyngeal and hypoglossal nerve) or surgery (accessory nerve), or a combination of both.

- Neck fibrosis:

  - Radiation therapy produces many changes at the cellular level, even to healthy tissues. A cumulative effect of these changes is the development of soft-tissue fibrosis:
    o This can lead to decreased range of motion, pain, and muscle spasms.
    o Soft-tissue fibrosis in the neck also can lead to carotid bulb dysfunction and cranial nerve palsies.

  - Lymphedema may occur after radiation and can be symptomatic. A specialized physical therapist can teach daily massage techniques.

Risk Reduction/Early Detection

- Refer to Chapter 5 to obtain cancer screening guidelines and algorithms on breast, cervical, colorectal, endometrial, ovarian, liver, lung, and skin cancers and HPV vaccinations
- Smoking cessation:

  - Lung cancer screenings for those with a history of smoking; refer to *Screening for Lung Cancer: Systematic Review to Update the U.S. Preventive Services Task Force Recommendation*

- Diet and weight management
- Exercise and activity
- Limit alcohol

Psychosocial Health and Functioning

- Distress:

  - Refer to the MD Anderson clinical practice algorithm, Distress Screening and Psychosocial Management of Adult Cancer Patients (available at www.mdanderson.org).
  - This section focuses on psychosocial concerns specific to survivors of head and neck cancers.
  - Some late effects of head and neck cancer treatments can lead to substantial distress and social isolation:
    o Dysphagia can lead to slow and/or noisy eating, causing embarrassment and social isolation.
    o Some patients need to use a percutaneous endoscopic gastrostomy feeding tube for nutrition and may not be able to take in food by mouth. These patients may be embarrassed to use their feeding tube in public and may not be able to participate in social functions during which eating is the main activity.
    o A consultation with a body image therapist may be warranted when social issues arise. If a body image therapist is not available, a psychotherapist, psychologist, or psychiatrist may be considered.

- Relationship issues:

  - Inquire about family status, peer relationships, participation in community and social activities, and communication with healthcare professionals.
  - Promote communication with parents/spouse/partner/siblings.
  - Provide information about psychosocial support and behavioral services:
    o Support groups and social and recreational programs:
    — Local support groups may be available.
    — Webwhisper.org hosts an online support group for patients with laryngeal cancer.
    — The Oral Cancer Foundation is a support group for patients with oral cancer.
  - Refer to social services.

- Body image issues:

  - Visible scars and reconstructive tissue can lead to body image disorders.
  - Head and neck cancer survivors may experience some degree of swallowing dysfunction ranging from prolonged eating time to a complete inability to orally ingest nutrition or hydration:
    - o This dysfunction can initially lead to embarrassment and ultimately lead to social isolation.
  - Laryngeal cancer survivors may experience alterations in, or the complete loss of, their ability to speak:
    - o This can be especially stressful for those who were comfortable speaking in public.

- Access to health care services (refer to Chapter 2: Tools for Clinicians):

  - Some head and neck cancer survivors will benefit from speech rehabilitative services.
  - Patients who experience decreased neck and shoulder range of motion may benefit from physical therapy.
  - Therapeutic massage may be useful for patients experiencing soft-tissue fibrosis of the neck.
  - Acupuncture may provide relief for patients with xerostomia.

- Employment status/financial stressors: Financial burden is associated with poor patient outcomes and increased mortality risk:

  - Employment issues:
    - o Cancer treatment effects such as speech and swallowing problems can interfere with survivors' ability to perform certain types of work, particularly tasks involving communication:
      - — Prepare patients for possible financial challenges they may encounter as they return to work, such as a decrease in workload or hours.
      - — Patients may need to consider transitioning from a full-time position to a part-time role.
      - — Patients may need to request a different job position.
    - o Encourage patients to ask their employer about available types of assistance such as an employee assistance program.
    - o Consider a social worker referral so patients can receive information about government assistance.
    - o Help patients fill out Family and Medical Leave Act forms or provide a supporting letter that details any job restrictions or limitations.
  - Financial stressors:
    - o Financial burdens related to treatment costs can continue throughout the survivorship period.
    - o Older cancer survivors with limited incomes are especially susceptible to financial burden because of their inability to work or forced retirement.

o Assess for financial issues.
o If needed, provide lists of local, state, or national financial assistance services and/or organizations.
o Link qualified survivors to Medicaid, Social Security, and/or disability insurance and/or transportation services.
o Consider referral to a social worker or a case manager.

CLINICAL VIGNETTE

SLC is a nonsmoking, married, and employed 53-year-old Caucasian male diagnosed with oropharyngeal squamous cell carcinoma 5 years ago. Prior to diagnosis, he developed a painless right neck mass. A cervical neck ultrasound confirmed lymphadenopathy and FNA biopsy revealed squamous cell carcinoma positive for high-risk HPV via in-situ hybridization. His oncologist discovered his primary site of tumor was in the base of tongue. He underwent definitive treatment with 60 Gy of intensity modulated radiation therapy divided into 30 daily fractions along with weekly Cisplatin. An 8-week posttherapy restaging work-up revealed that SLC had no evidence of disease.

Questions

1. Posttreatment, SLC should be monitored for
   A. Hearing changes
   B. Hypothyroidism
   C. Dental caries or osteoradionecrosis of the jaw
   D. All of the above
   E. B and C

2. How often should you check this patient's thyroid functions?
   A. Annually
   B. Only until replacement is needed, then no more
   C. At least annually and if he develops symptoms

3. What intervention has been shown to benefit postradiation dental health?
   A. Four times daily teeth brushing
   B. Daily use of fluoride gel dental trays
   C. Prophylactic total mouth extraction of unhealthy and healthy teeth
   D. Using an electronic toothbrush

4. True/False—SLC's diagnosis of an HPV(+) squamous cell oropharyngeal cancer proves marital infidelity.
   A. True
   B. False

5. Given SLC's diagnosis, which members of his family should get the HPV vaccine?
   A. All members
   B. His partner
   C. His children age 11 to 26
   D. All children age 11 to 26

Answers

1. D
SLC received radiation therapy to the oropharynx and cervical lymph nodes. He also received concurrent Cisplatin, which is known for its ototoxic side-effects. His thyroid gland was within the radiation field and should therefore be monitored for acute and chronic dysfunction. His teeth were also within the field of radiation, particularly his mandibular teeth, and therefore will require monitoring for caries due to the loss of protective enamel.

2. C
SLC's thyroid gland is at risk for acute and chronic dysfunction due to the radiation therapy. His levels should be checked at least annually, and should be checked if he develops any symptoms of hypothyroidism. The provider should be familiar with both immediate and long-term signs and symptoms of hypothyroidism.

3. B
Radiation therapy and loss of saliva cause break down of the protective enamel layer of teeth. Daily use of fluoride trays helps to strengthen irradiated teeth and avoid dental injuries. Radiation also decreases microvasculature to the bone and patients are at risk for osteoradionecrosis. Healthy teeth do not need to be extracted prior to radiation. It is not recommended to have dental extractions after radiation.

4. B
Although there may have been marital infidelity, this diagnosis does not specifi-cally prove it. It is important for the provider to understand that the actual HPV exposure and infection took place decades prior to the development into a malignancy. It is important for the provider to understand the pathophysiology of HPV infection.

5. D
All children qualify for the HPV vaccine at the age of 11 up until 26. The HPV vaccine prevents cancer if given prior to HPV exposure, therefore early vaccination is encouraged. Patients with HPV related cancers have likely had exposure decades before developing disease and are not considered infectious. Partners do not need vaccination as they likely have already been exposed and vaccination will not be effective.

RECOMMENDED READINGS

Cohen EE, LaMonte SJ, Erb NL, et al. American cancer society head and neck cancer survivorship care guideline. *CA Cancer J Clin.* 2016;66(3):203–239.

Foxhall LE, Rodriguez MA. *Advances in Cancer Survivorship Management.* New York, NY: Springer; 2015.

Humphrey L, Deffebach M, Pappas M, et al. *Screening for Lung Cancer: Systematic Review to Update the U.S. Preventive Services Task Force Recommendation (Evidence Syntheses, No 105).* Rockville, Maryland: Agency for Healthcare Research and Quality; 2013. Available at: https://www.ncbi.nlm.nih.gov/sites/books/NBK154610.

Hutcheson KA, Lewis CM. Head and neck cancer survivorship management. In: Foxhall LE, Rodriguez MA, eds. *Advances in Cancer Survivorship Management*: New York, NY: Springer; 2015:145–166.

Mercado G, Adelstein DJ, Saxton JP, et al. Hypothyroidism. *Cancer.* 2001;92(11): 2892–2897.

Miller MC, Shuman AG. Survivorship in head and neck cancer: a primer. *JAMA Otolaryngol Head Neck Surg.* 2016;142(10):1002–1008.

Siegel RL, Miller KD, Jemal A. Cancer statistics, 2015. *CA Cancer J Clin.* 2015;65(1):5–29.

Viens LJ. Human papillomavirus–associated cancers—United States, 2008–2012. *Morb Mortal Wkly Rep.* 2016;65(26):661–666.

Lymphoma Survivorship Care

Maria Alma Rodriguez
Ellen Mullen
Haleigh Mistry

CLINICAL PEARLS

- For this group of survivors, the examination must focus on lymph node characteristics. Note the number, size, and location.

- Patients who have had mediastinal radiation will be at risk for premature coronary artery disease and sclerosis of the cardiac valves. To prevent acceleration of arteriosclerosis, monitor lipid levels and treat high cholesterol levels with statins.

- The shingles vaccine may be considered if a patient's immunoglobulins and white cell populations (including monocytes and lymphocytes) are within defined limits. However, live virus vaccines are contraindicated in patients who have immunoglobulin deficiencies or a decreased total white cell count or decreased absolute lymphocyte count.

LYMPHOMA EPIDEMIOLOGY AND SURVIVORSHIP CARE

- Background:

  - Most common hematologic cancer
  - The World Health Organization (WHO) classification system, released in 2001, has proven consistent and reliable with schema based on four characteristics: clinical features, morphology, immunophenotype, and genetics
  - According to the WHO classification, lymphoma is a heterogeneous disease with more than 30 subtypes
  - Two major distinct groups: patients with Hodgkin's lymphoma (HL) and non-HL (NHL)
  - In general, incidence rates for lymphoma are decreasing but vary by subtype
  - Lymphoma is most common in people ages 65 and older, but subtype varies by age
  - Precursor B-cell lymphoblastic leukemias/lymphomas are most common among children ages 14 and younger

■ Non-Hispanic whites have the best survival rates; Hispanic white, Asian, and Asian Pacific Islanders have middle survival rates, and blacks have the worst survival across all lymphoma subtypes.

■ Survival rates are better when diagnosis occurs at a younger age with limited disease stage and without B symptoms or an HIV/AIDs diagnosis.

■ Death rates for lymphomas have been decreasing for 4 decades as treatment modalities improve.

• The two most common lymphoid neoplasms:

■ HL and NHL:
   o Incidence:
      — There are four groups of HLs; nodular sclerosis HL is the most common.
      — Among NHL groups, diffuse large B-cell lymphoma (DLBCL) and follicular lymphoma (FL) are the most common subtypes.
         a. DLBCLs grow more quickly; FLs grow more slowly but may be aggressive depending upon cell size.
   o Survival:
      — Survival rates vary greatly by disease stage and subtype.
      — For HL, the 5-year survival rate is 86%, and the 10-year rate is 80%.
      — For NHL, the 5-year survival rate is 70%, and the 10-year rate is 60%.
      — B-cell lymphoma 5-year survival rates range between 78% and 92%.

• Clinical tools to guide care for lymphoma survivors:

■ Eligibility criteria for transition of patients with DLBCL to survivorship care (refer to Figure 14.1).

■ Eligibility criteria for transition of patients with HL to survivorship care (refer to Figure 14.2).

■ Algorithms for other types of lymphomas:
   o Follicular B-cell lymphoma for Stages I or II
   o Peripheral T-cell lymphoma

DISEASE SURVEILLANCE

• Medical history and physical examination:

■ General examination:
   o For this group of survivors, the examination must focus on lymph node characteristics. Note the number, size, and location.
   o Ask the survivor if he or she has experienced changes such as acute pruritus, night sweats, unplanned weight loss, or painless lymphadenopathy.
   o Review the patient's vital signs and note blood pressure, body mass index, and pulse. Refer to the section on cardiovascular system examinations.

■ Head and neck examination:

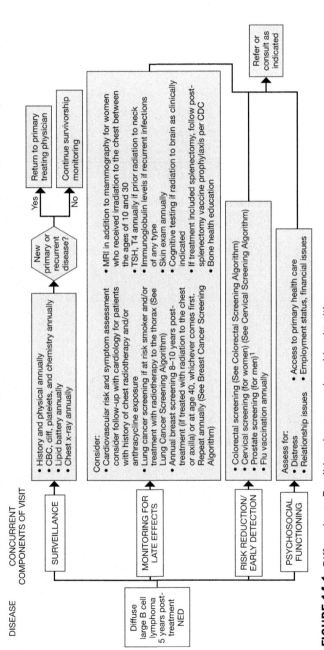

FIGURE 14.1 Diffuse large B-cell lymphoma survivorship algorithm.

NED, no evidence of disease; [1]Based on American Cancer Society Prostate Cancer Screening Guidelines. *Source:* Copyright 2015 The University of Texas MD Anderson Cancer Center.

170

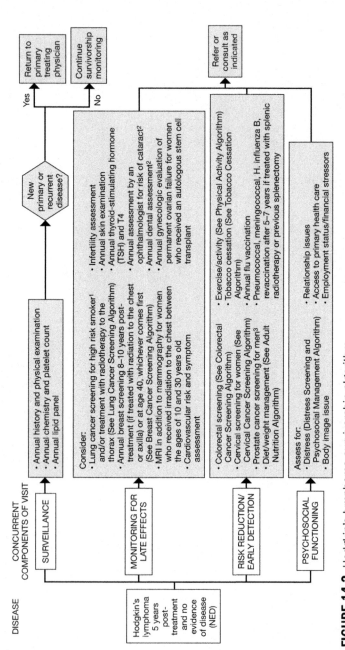

FIGURE 14.2 Hodgkin's lymphoma survivorship algorithm.

[1]High-risk smoker: age 55–80 years old, greater than or equal to 30 pack per year smoking history, current or previous smoker; [2]For patients who received an autologous stem cell transplant; [3]Based on American Cancer Society Prostate Cancer Screening Guidelines. *Source:* Copyright 2017 The University of Texas MD Anderson Cancer Center.

- o Examine lymphatic nodes in preauricular, submandibular, postauricular, occipital, and cervical neck areas. If any enlarged nodes (>1.5 cm) are noted, a biopsy either by core needle procedure or excision is recommended.
- o For patients who have had radiation to head/neck regions and smokers, perform an oral examination to assess for ulcers or leukoplakia, decay, oral dryness, visible masses, or mucosal changes. If changes are noted, refer to an appropriate dental or ENT specialist.
- o Thyroid palpation for nodules/masses: If palpable nodules/masses are found, recommend thyroid ultrasound. Fine-needle aspiration or biopsy of palpable masses may be indicated based on ultrasound results.
- o Fundus examination: Accelerated development of cataracts is associated with steroids (used in many lymphoma regimens) and orbital irradiation. If a patient has diabetes, refer to an ophthalmologist for a yearly complete eye examination.
- ■ Thoracic examination:
  - o Examine supraclavicular, infraclavicular, and axillary nodal sites; if enlargement is noted, further evaluation is recommended.
  - o Lung auscultation: If the patient is a smoker or has a history of asthma, carefully note and document rales, wheezes, or rhonchi:
    — If patients have new-onset shortness of breath with minimal exertion, review chest x-ray findings for indications of pleural effusion, lung infiltrates, or new hilar or mediastinal nodes. Please note cancer screening guidelines for smokers, which include thin-slice chest CT.
    — A referral to a pulmonary or cardiology specialist may be indicated if findings are abnormal. Patients with bleomycin exposure are at risk for decreased diffusing lung capacity; obtain pulmonary function tests if new symptoms arise.
- ■ Cardiovascular examination:
  - o Perform heart auscultation to assess for murmur, gallop, rub, or an irregular rhythm or rate. If patients have had mediastinal radiation, premature sclerosis of valves may occur but it is very unusual to develop late pericarditis. If a new-onset murmur is noted, recommend an echocardiogram.
  - o Perform auscultation of carotids for bruits. Patients who have had radiation to neck nodes are at higher risk for carotid artery stenosis related to arteriosclerosis; if a bruit is present, obtain a carotid Doppler examination.
  - o Examine pulses and cardiac rhythm for irregularities; an electrocardiogram is recommended if a new rhythm abnormality is detected or if there is a new or unexplained rapid or slow pulse.
  - o Examine for pedal edema; this nonspecific finding may be prompted by a number of conditions including excess sodium intake, renal dysfunction, early signs of cardiac failure, and poor peripheral vascular circulation, among others. Correlate with other physical findings and laboratory studies if edema is present.
- ■ Abdominal examination:
  - o Examine the liver and spleen; splenomegaly or hepatomegaly may signal lymphoma recurrence. If hepatomegaly is noted in patients with a history of

hepatitis B or C and if liver function test findings are elevated, obtain viral titers to evaluate for reactivation. Evaluate with liver ultrasound because patients are at higher risk for hepatoma if they have had hepatitis B.

o Palpate for any new masses or signs/symptoms of pain:

— If there are palpable masses or new-onset pain, CT evaluation is needed. If there is new-onset blood in stool or changes in stool, refer to a gastrointestinal specialist for evaluation.

— If there is a history of radiation to the abdomen or pelvis or a familial history of colon cancer, the patient may be at higher risk for secondary colon cancer.

■ Musculoskeletal examination:

o Assess for muscle wasting in radiation areas.

o Assess for joint deformities or swelling; there may be accelerated degenerative changes if the joint is within a radiation port.

o Observe for extremity size asymmetry:

— Patients may develop unilateral swelling of extremities attributable to new venous thrombi or lymphedema.

— If there is unilateral unexplained swelling, obtain a Doppler of the extremity to rule out thrombus.

— If there is no thrombus and lymphedema is suspected, refer to a physical therapy specialist for lymphedema management.

■ Neurological examination:

o Assess for asymmetry in muscle movement or strength:

— Patients with history of radiation to the cervical spine may develop Lhermitte syndrome.

— An MRI of the brain and/or spine may be indicated if there are new neurological changes or symptoms.

o Deep tendon reflexes may be lost in distal lower extremities secondary to peripheral neuropathy; this is common if a patient has been treated with vinca alkaloids (vincristine, vinorelbine), taxanes (taxol, taxotere), and proteosome inhibitors (bortezomib, lenalidomide).

■ Skin examination:

o Examine areas of sun or radiation exposure.

o Note any new or unusual dark moles, scaly lesions, or multiple atypical nevi. Refer to a dermatologist to assess these findings.

o Observe for petechial lesions; a complete blood count (CBC) with platelets must be ordered if there are new-onset petechial lesions. Order international normalized ratio, prothrombin time, and partial thromboplastin time labs if unexplained new ecchymosis occurs.

o Assess for rashes or vesicles; patients with a history of chicken pox are at risk for reactivation (shingles).

o Patients with persistent skin rashes should undergo biopsy to rule out a secondary lymphoma or autoimmune or infectious rash etiologies.

■ Pelvic examination:

o Examine inguinal and femoral nodes; if any enlargement exceeds 1.5 cm, biopsy is recommended.

o If premenopausal women experience acute pelvic pain or bleeding, loss of menses, or palpable uterine enlargement, a pregnancy test is indicated, and evaluation by a gynecologist is needed.

o Recommend a fertility evaluation and gynecological care for women; men should see a urologist.

o If pelvic masses are detected upon examination, CT studies are indicated. Pregnancy tests should be done prior to CT studies in premenopausal women.

- Laboratory tests:

  - CBC with differential and platelet count to assess for anemia, thrombocytopenia, or leukocyte population changes
  - Chemistry profile to monitor for vital organ function (liver, renal) and nutritional/metabolic parameters (glucose, albumin, total protein, etc.)
  - Immunoglobulin levels to assess for recurrent infection of any type and monoclonal gammopathy and to monitor recovery of B-cell function
  - Thyroid-stimulating hormone and T4 annually if the patient has had neck irradiation to monitor for hypothyroidism
  - Vitamin D level to check for deficiencies that may impact bone health
  - Lipid profile to monitor for high low-density lipoprotein (LDL) and low high-density lipoprotein (HDL)
  - Prostate-specific antigen to monitor/screen for prostate abnormalities

- Chest x-ray is performed to detect or monitor:

  - Changes in mediastinal and hilar nodes
  - Bone density changes or new bone lesions
  - Lung parenchymal nodules, masses, or parenchymal infiltrates
  - Pleural effusions or masses
  - Heart size changes and aorta and/or coronary calcifications
  - Soft-tissue masses in the upper torso, axilla, or supraclavicular spaces

MONITORING FOR LATE EFFECTS

- Cardiovascular risk and symptom assessment:

  - Patients who have had mediastinal radiation will be at risk for premature coronary artery disease and sclerosis of the cardiac valves. To prevent acceleration of arteriosclerosis, monitor lipid levels and treat high cholesterol levels with statins.
  - Hypertension and diabetes should be managed to prevent exacerbation of cardiac disease risks. If patients describe new-onset chest pain or dyspnea, a cardiac evaluation is recommended to rule out ischemia.
  - If a new-onset murmur is noted, an echocardiogram is recommended. There is controversy regarding optimal frequency of echocardiogram studies for patients who have received anthracyclines and/or mediastinal radiation. Patients should have pretreatment baseline and posttreatment echocardiograms, with repeat studies at regular intervals and at any time new signs or symptoms of cardiac insufficiency develop.

- Patients who have had radiation to neck nodes are at elevated risk for carotid artery stenosis related to arteriosclerosis; if a bruit is involved, obtain carotid Doppler examinations.
- Cardiac arrhythmias may manifest years after radiation and chemotherapy treatment.
- An electrocardiogram is recommended if a new rhythm abnormality is detected or if there is a new or unexplained rapid or slow pulse.

- Lung function and cancer screening:

  - Patients who are active smokers or those who have lung radiation exposure from mediastinal or upper body nodal radiation are at risk for secondary primary lung cancers.
  - Smoking cessation is strongly urged for active smokers. If a patient has received bleomycin (as part of the ABVD [Adriamycin, bleomycin, vinblastine, dacarbazine] regimen for HL), they are at risk for late pulmonary fibrosis and a secondary decrease in diffusing lung capacity.
  - Obtain pulmonary function tests if progressive dyspnea symptoms develop. A pulmonary consultation and rehabilitation may be appropriate for some patients, and caution is urged for those who need to undergo surgery with general anesthesia and oxygen supplementation because pulmonary fibrosis secondary to bleomycin use may worsen.
  - Patients with a history of asbestos exposure will be at risk for mesothelioma. A yearly chest x-ray is recommended, and findings that suggest new lung masses will merit further workup to rule out malignancy or atypical infections.

- Oral cavity late effects:

  - For patients who have had radiation to head/neck regions and all smokers, there is risk for secondary oropharyngeal malignancies.
  - Oral dryness also may occur, although newer radiation techniques have substantially decreased this side effect. Patients need to drink water frequently to moisten their mouth, and artificial saliva may be helpful.
  - There may be acceleration of dental decay; as a result, fluoride gel prophylaxis is recommended. Patients need to have dental cleanings on a frequent and regular basis and be monitored by their dentist.

- Orbital examination:

  - Cataract risk is associated with steroid use (used in many lymphoma regimens) and orbital irradiation.
  - Eye dryness may develop and may be exacerbated if a patient has diabetes. Artificial tears are recommended.
  - These patients should be referred to an ophthalmologist for a yearly complete eye examination.

- Endocrine system evaluation:

  - Thyroid examination:
    o Patients may develop hypothyroidism if they have received radiation to the upper thorax/mediastinum or head and neck region. This may occur promptly after therapy or many years later.

- o New generations of chemotherapy agents such as the tyrosine kinase inhibitors and immune-modulating therapies such as nivolumab are known to cause disruption of thyroid function, so patients who are exposed to these treatments may need lifelong monitoring and hormone replacement therapy.
- ▪ Diabetes:
  - o Steroids exacerbate diabetes and can precipitate new-onset diabetes in patients who have metabolic syndrome at the onset of chemotherapy. In this setting, diabetes usually persists after chemotherapy ends.
  - o These patients require appropriate care and monitoring for diabetes management (hemoglobin A1C testing and renal, pedal, and ophthalmology care).

- Sexual function assessment:

  - ▪ Chemotherapy usually suppresses sexual hormones, and premature menopause onset usually occurs in women older than age 30 when they receive chemotherapy.
  - ▪ Men may experience a drop in testosterone hormone levels with a decrease in libido and possible erectile dysfunction. Both men and women may need hormone replacement therapies after lymphoma treatment, and patients should be referred as indicated to urology or gynecology services, respectively.
  - ▪ Consider a sexual counseling referral if sexual function impairment is perceived by a patient and/or his or her partner as a substantial problem in their relationship.

- Infertility assessment:

  - ▪ Refer to MD Anderson's clinical practice algorithms, Fertility Preservation to Cancer Treatment, Fertility Sparing Treatment, and Pregnancy Screening (available at www.mdanderson.org).
  - ▪ Educate patients about treatment-related infertility risk. Chemotherapies used in the treatment of lymphoma such as alkylating agents can damage maturing sperm and oocytes. Pelvic radiation or total-body irradiation can cause ovarian and testicular dysfunction.
  - ▪ Recommend fertility preservation for patients of reproductive age (premenopausal females and males of any age who wish to preserve sperm to potentially father future children).

RISK REDUCTION/EARLY DETECTION

- This section focuses on risk reduction specific to lymphoma survivors:

  - ▪ Refer to Chapter 5 for screening guidelines and algorithms on breast, cervical, colorectal, endometrial, ovarian, liver, lung, and skin cancers and human papilloma virus (HPV) vaccinations.

- Correlation between lymphoma survivors and secondary malignancies:

  - ▪ Surveillance, Epidemiology, and End Results findings: Patients with NHL who received radiotherapy are at elevated risk for breast cancer, sarcomas, and mesothelioma (SIR 1.14).

- Lung cancer screening guidelines for lymphoma survivors: Screening is needed for patients who:
  - Have a history of mediastinal radiation
  - Are current smokers
  - Have a 30-pack-year smoking history
- Breast screening:
  - Screening via bilateral mammography is needed for 8 to 10 years posttreatment (if a patient has been treated with radiation to the chest or axilla) or at age 40, whichever comes first
  - Repeat annually
- Skin screening:
  - Risk factors specific to lymphoma survivors:
    o History of HL or NHL attributable to immunosuppressive therapy
    o Cancer risk is increased in the radiation treatment field after therapy ends
- Vaccinations:
  - A yearly flu vaccine is recommended for those who are not allergic to the vaccine, and a pneumococcal vaccination also is recommended with a booster every 5 years.
  - Patients who have had monoclonal antibodies or other immune therapies that may lead to immune suppression or deficiencies are at risk for reactivation of viral infections such as herpes zoster and hepatitis B and atypical infections.
  - The shingles vaccine may be considered if a patient's immunoglobulins and white cell populations (including monocytes and lymphocytes) are within defined limits. However, live virus vaccines are contraindicated in patients who have immunoglobulin deficiencies or a decreased total white cell count or decreased absolute lymphocyte count.
  - Patients who have had splenectomy are at risk for infections of encapsulated bacteria such as *Streptococcus*, *Pneumococcus*, and *Meningococcus*, which can be fatal for this population. Immunizations should have been administered prior to the splenectomy.
  - The Centers for Disease Control and Prevention recommends periodic boosters postsplenectomy.

PSYCHOSOCIAL HEALTH AND FUNCTIONING

- Distress:
  - Refer to the MD Anderson clinical practice algorithm, Distress Screening and Psychosocial Management of Adult Cancer Patients (available at www.mdanderson.org). This section focuses on psychosocial concerns specific to lymphoma survivors.
  - For patients who have had central nervous system (CNS) lymphoma, a neurocognitive assessment should have been performed before and after treatment; repeat these assessments when changes in cognitive patterns are reported by family members or observed upon examination.

- Brain MRI is indicated when people develop behavioral changes that are atypical, abnormal, or out of the ordinary to rule out CNS lymphoma recurrence versus new vascular, infectious, or other organic causes.

- Relationship issues:

  - Inquire about family status, peer relationships, participation in community and social activities, and communication with healthcare professionals.
  - Promote communication between parents/spouse/partners/siblings.
  - Provide information about psychosocial support and behavioral services, age-appropriate support groups, and social and recreational programs.
  - Refer to Social Services.
  - Refer to age-appropriate peer support groups.

- Body image issues:

  - Alopecia:
    - Hair loss can result from radiation, targeted, and hormonal therapies and chemotherapy.
    - Hair loss from cancer treatment can be an emotionally challenging experience that affects body image and quality of life.
    - Encourage patient to talk about their feelings and experience with friends, family members, and counselors.
    - Provide information about medications for hair growth.
    - Provide a prescription for scalp prosthesis (hairpiece or wig). Insurance companies may cover the cost, and these purchases also qualify as tax-deductible medical expenses.
    - Link survivors to cancer centers or community organizations at which they can obtain free or loaner wigs or hairpieces.
  - Lymphedema:
    - Surgical resections of lymph nodes and/or radiation therapy are two major risk factors associated with lymphedema.
    - Chronic lymphedema usually occurs 18 to 24 months postsurgery but also may appear years later.
    - Lymphedema treatment involves preventing infection, reducing tissue load, and avoiding pressure changes.
    - Refer to physical therapy or a lymphedema clinic if necessary.
    - Refer to lymphedema support groups if necessary.
    - Refer to psychiatry for counseling if necessary.

- Employment status/financial stressors:

  - Employment issues:
    - Financial burden is associated with poor patient outcomes and increased mortality risk.
    - Cancer treatment effects such as chronic fatigue, pain, neuropathy, and cognitive and sensory impairments can interfere with survivors' abilities to perform

certain types of work. Prepare patients about possible challenges they may face as they go back to work such as decreased workload or hours, transition from full time to part time, or position changes.

o Encourage patients to ask their employer about types of available assistance.

o Refer to a social worker so patients can receive information about available government assistance.

o Help patients fill out Family and Medical Leave Act forms or provide a supportive letter regarding job restrictions/limitations.

- Financial issues:

  ▪ The financial burden associated with treatment costs can persist throughout the survivorship period. This burden poses a problem for older cancer survivors with limited incomes and inability to work. These survivors may be forced to retire:
    o Assess for financial issues.
    o Provide lists of local or national services or organizations such as the Lymphoma and Leukemia Society.
    o Link qualified survivors to Medicaid, Social Security, and/or disability insurance/transportation programs.

  ▪ Refer to a social worker or case manager.

CLINICAL VIGNETTE

JMR is a 60-year-old woman who learned she had HL when she developed a mediastinal mass at age 20. At the time of her diagnosis, the standard-of-care staging procedure included laparotomy with abdominal lymph node sampling and splenectomy. She received pneumococcal and meningococcal vaccines before her splenectomy. Her disease stage was IIA, and she was treated with radiation to a mantle field.

1. Posttreatment, this patient should be closely monitored for
   A. Thyroid function studies at least yearly or at any time she develops symptoms suggesting hypothyroidism
   B. Skin problems, particularly within the radiation port
   C. Dental caries and dry mouth
   D. All the above
   E. Only A and B

2. The most serious immediate posttreatment malignancy risk for this patient is
   A. HL recurrence
   B. Skin cancers within the radiation port
   C. Breast cancer

   D. Thyroid cancer
   E. None of the above

3. JMR arrives at your clinic as a new patient. You should pay particular attention to her
   A. Smoking history
   B. Vaccination history
   C. Date of last colonoscopy
   D. All of the above
   E. Only A and B

4. A life-threatening potential late treatment effect that is particularly concerning when considering this patient's age is
   A. Cardiac valve and coronary arterial sclerosis
   B. Bone density loss
   C. Renal function decline
   D. Pulmonary function impairment
   E. Depression

Answers

1. D

All of the listed problems are reported complications associated with mantle radiation. Loss of thyroid function may occur at any time postradiation as an immediate radiation thyroiditis event or as a slowly declining process that may manifest many years later. The skin within the radiation port should be protected against sun damage and observed for suspicious changes or lesions. Patients should not tan artificially and are advised to wear protective clothing. The design of the mantle fields at the time this patient was treated would have had allowed substantial radiation exposure to the salivary glands and mouth dryness would occur, with a secondary effect of accelerated dental caries. Patients should use fluoride rinse solutions to prevent this problem.

2. A

The 3- to 5-year time frame immediately after treatment poses highest risk for HL recurrence, although for patients with Stage IIA disease treated with radiation only, overall risk for relapse is low. All other malignancies listed can arise as secondary malignancies. Breast cancer, in particular, is a concern for this patient because she received radiation at a relatively young age, and radiation port design techniques would have exposed her breast tissue to radiation. However, second primary cancers usually do not pose immediate risk; risks begin to rise 5 to 10 years after treatment ends.

3. D

Because this patient is now 60 years old, her lung cancer risk as a smoker will be exacerbated by past radiation treatment. She must be counseled to attend smoking cessation programs or receive medical therapy to help her to stop smoking. Because she has had a splenectomy, she is particularly susceptible to bacterial infections, especially encapsulated organisms. She should be advised regarding Centers for Disease Control and Prevention recommendations for vaccination boosters. At this patient's age, she should have had at least one colonoscopy because risk for secondary malignancies is increased in long-term Hodgkin's disease survivors.

4. A

Radiation in a mantle field port exposed this patient's heart to radiation. Modern port design and dose-delivery techniques are more focused and are associated with less scatter, but cardiac tissue continues to pose risk. Cardiovascular disease is one of the two leading causes of death among Hodgkin's disease survivors (the other being death attributable to cancer). For patients with prior radiation to the mediastinum, it is very important to track hypertension, hyperlipidemias, diabetes, and body mass index. Although bone density loss also is an important and recognized effect of radiation to the axial skeleton that warrants treatment, it is not an imminent life-threatening problem. Renal function decline is not an anticipated late effect of radiation to the upper body. Pulmonary function impairment may occur, particularly if a patient is a smoker, but often this impairment is not life threatening. Depression and anxiety may be long lasting for some patients despite many years of remission. Again, support and referral to mental health specialists is appropriate if these problems persist.

RECOMMENDED READINGS

Al-Hamadani M, Habermann TM, Cerhan JR, et al. Non-Hodgkin lymphoma subtype distribution, geodemographic patterns, and survival in the US: longitudinal analysis of the National Cancer Data Base from 1998 to 2011. *Am J Hematol*. 2015;90(9):790–795.

Beckjord EB, Arora NK, Bellizzi K, et al. Sexual well-being among survivors of non-Hodgkin lymphoma. *Oncol Nurs Forum*. 2011;38(5):E351–E359.

Denlinger CS, Ligibel JA, Are M, et al. NCCN guidelines insights: survivorship, version 1.2016. *J Natl Compr Canc Netw*. 2016;14(6):715–724.

Flowers CR, Armitage JO. A decade of progress in lymphoma: advances and continuing challenges. *Clin Lymphoma Myeloma and Leuk*. 2010;10(6):414–423.

Han X, Kilfoy B, Zheng T, et al. Lymphoma survival patterns by WHO subtype in the United States, 1973–2003. *Cancer Causes Control*. 2008;19(8):841–858.

Jones SM, Ziebell R, Walker R, et al. Association of worry about cancer to benefit finding and functioning in long-term cancer survivors. *Support Care Cancer*. 2017;25(5):1417–1422. doi:10.1007/s00520-016-3537-z

Leak A, Mayer DK, Smith S. Quality of life domains among non-Hodgkin lymphoma survivors: an integrative literature review. *Leuk Lymphoma*. 2011;52(6):972–985.

Melisko ME, Narus JB. Sexual function in cancer survivors: updates to the NCCN guidelines for survivorship. *J Natl Compr Canc Netw.* 2016;14(suppl 5):685–689.

Morton LM, Wang SS, Devesa SS, et al. Lymphoma incidence patterns by WHO subtype in the United States, 1992–2001. *Blood.* 2006;107(1):265–276.

Naughton MJ, Weaver KE. Physical and mental health among cancer survivors: considerations for long-term care and quality of life. *N C Med J.* 2014;75(4):283–286.

Nekhlyudov L, Walker R, Ziebell R, et al. Cancer survivors' experiences with insurance, finances, and employment: results from a multisite study. *J Cancer Surviv.* 2016;10(6):1104–1111.

Rodriguez MA, Ballas L, Simar K. Hematologic cancer survivorship management: lymphoma. In: Foxhall LE and Rodriguez MA, eds. *Advances in Cancer Survivorship Management.* New York, NY: Springer; 2015:201–218.

Walker E, Martins A, Aldiss S, et al. Psychosocial interventions for adolescents and young adults diagnosed with cancer during adolescence: a critical review. *J Adolesc Young Adult Oncol.* 2016;5(4):310–321.

15

Survivorship Care for Recipients of Hematopoietic Stem Cell Transplantation

Karen Stolar
Alison Gulbis
Amin Alousi

CLINICAL PEARLS

- Hematopoietic stem cell transplantation (HSCT) may be indicated when treatment history clearly reveals resistant, progressing, or recurrent disease after one or more treatment regimens is administered.

- Post-HSCT maintenance therapy with disease-specific drugs may be offered to HSCT recipients to improve long-term disease-free survival and may involve varying durations ranging from months to years.

- Survivors with ongoing immunosuppressive medication requirements may need more frequent monitoring, and the HSCT team typically will provide direction.

A UNIQUE AT-RISK POPULATION

Patients who undergo HSCT frequently are not seen in primary care practices and represent a unique subset of cancer survivors. These survivors are at risk for life-altering late effects of disease and treatment attributed to the complex interactions of comorbidities, prior transplant-related and posttransplant maintenance treatments, immunodeficiency, peri- and early posttransplant medical events, and social support and lifestyle. During the early years after treatment, disease relapse and infection are the most common causes of morbidity and mortality.

Although this chapter focuses on problematic late effects, it is important to note that most HSCT survivors relate positive, forward momentum during the years after HSCT. They commonly endorse good quality of life and show heroic coping and adaptation in seemingly impossible situations. They display increasingly improved health and a new attention to preserving their health through lifestyle improvements. They describe a sense of personal growth, improved family and social relationships, deepened spirituality, and an overall sense of well-being. Take the time to listen to the story of each journey at least once during your relationship with each HSCT survivor. HSCT can be an affirming and therapeutic intervention for a survivor and a humbling and renewing experience for healthcare providers.

GENERAL STEM CELL TRANSPLANTATION BACKGROUND

HSCT most commonly is used to treat specific oncologic, blood, and autoimmune disorders and severe metabolism disorders. Indications for HSCT include diseases for which standard chemotherapy, radiation therapy, and/or immunotherapy are unlikely to provide long-term disease survival. HSCT also may be indicated when treatment history clearly reveals resistant, progressing, or recurrent disease after one or more treatment regimens is administered.

- Diseases for which HSCT commonly is used as treatment include acute, chronic, and secondary leukemia; myelodysplastic syndrome; myeloproliferative disorders; aplastic anemia; lymphomas; myelomas; and other blood disorders such as Fanconi anemia, Diamond–Blackfan anemia, and thalassemia; severe immunodeficiency disorders; neuroblastoma; testicular cancer; and severe disorders of metabolism and autoimmune diseases such as multiple sclerosis.
- The type of HSCT a patient receives depends upon his or her disease and associated risk characteristics, the patient's physical and functional health at the time of transplant, and donor availability. There are two general types of HSCT:
  - Autologous: The patient's own stem cells are collected and cryopreserved before he or she receives high-dose chemotherapy and/or radiation therapy. After completing the treatment regimen for disease control or cure, commonly referred to as the "conditioning regimen," the patient's own cells are reinfused to rescue him or her from the effects of the regimen's bone marrow destruction. The newly infused stem cells regrow the marrow and the ability to make hematopoietic stem cells to provide red and white blood cells and platelets.
  - Allogeneic: A donor provides stem cells. The patient receives chemotherapy and/or radiation therapy for disease control or cure. After completing the regimen, donor stem cells are infused to regrow the marrow and the ability to make hematopoietic stem cells to provide red and white blood cells and platelets. An allogeneic transplant also provides transplant recipients with an immunotherapy effect of donor graft versus "tumor":
    o Donors may be related or unrelated to a patient. A patient may receive a "less-than-perfect" match depending upon donor availability. The closest match available should be sought. Table 15.1 details donor types and associated relationships.
- The stem cell source used for HSCT is determined by donor availability, donor health, and patient disease and treatment history:
  - Bone marrow stem cell transplant: A procedure is performed in the operating room to aspirate a volume and a calculated number of bone marrow stem cells from an autologous or allogeneic donor.

TABLE 15.1 Donor Types

Donor Type	Relationship
Matched related donor	Sibling
Haploidentical donor	Parent or sibling
Matched unrelated donor	The donor has no relationship to the patient
Umbilical cord blood donor	Typically unrelated; may be related if a family member's cord blood stem cells are available or the patient's own cord blood cells are available. Adults may need two donors to provide cells depending upon the number of cells in each cord product

- Peripheral blood stem cell transplant: An apheresis procedure is performed on an autologous or allogeneic donor, which may take several hours for 1 to 3 days. A calculated number of peripheral blood stem cells is collected.
- Umbilical cord blood stem cell transplant: Umbilical cord blood stem cells are collected from the donor's umbilical cord at the time of birth. The cells are cryopreserved and stored in a cord blood stem cell bank until a patient in need is identified.

HSCT-SPECIFIC CONSIDERATIONS IN SURVIVORSHIP CARE

All of these factors are important when developing a long-term follow-up plan:

- Cancer diagnosis
- Disease treatment(s) that were administered before the patient was referred for a HSCT. Most HSCT recipients have received treatment with multiple chemotherapies, radiation therapies, and/or immunotherapies and possibly surgery before they come to a HSCT program for treatment
- Age at HSCT
- Comorbid conditions
- HSCT conditioning regimen, which is the chemotherapy and potential radiation therapy administered days prior to the hematopoietic stem cell infusion
- Type of HSCT donor (autologous or allogeneic)
- The source of stem cells the patient received (peripheral blood stem cells, marrow stem cells, or cord blood stem cells)
- Peri- and post-HSCT medical events, the most impactful being graft versus host disease (GVHD), which is an allogeneic HSCT complication
- Post-HSCT maintenance therapy with disease-specific drugs. This continuing therapy may be offered to selected HSCT recipients to improve long-term disease-free survival and may involve varying durations ranging from months to years
- Immune reconstitution, which includes engraftment of all cell lines, discontinuation of immunosuppressive medications, evaluation of humoral immune system function including splenic function and thymic function, and revaccination

GRAFT VERSUS HOST DISEASE

- GVHD is a complex immune-mediated reaction in which an allogeneic donor's immune system attacks the recipient's body in one or more organ systems:
  - GVHD may occur days to weeks, months, or years after allogeneic HSCT. It is less likely to occur more than 3 years after allogeneic HSCT.
  - Severity and duration of GVHD can lead to a cascade of serious, potentially life-threatening medical events and impact quality of life for the duration of life.
  - GVHD prophylaxis is initiated before allogeneic HSCT with medication alone or in combination:
    - Common GVHD prophylaxis regimens include cyclosporine, tacrolimus, mini-dose methotrexate, mycophenolate mofetil, sirolimus, and post-HSCT cyclophosphamide:
      — Because GVHD prophylaxis regimens are immunosuppressive, an HSCT recipient also receives bacterial, viral, and fungal prophylaxis medications while receiving GVHD prophylaxis or treatment.
      — GVHD prophylaxis regimens are discontinued by weaning the medication(s) in a planned pattern at a specified time. The weaning process is individualized to each HSCT recipient and guided by type of HSCT, development of GVHD, and disease status under the direction of the HSCT team.
      — Once GVHD prophylaxis is discontinued, bacterial, viral, and fungal prophylaxis usually is discontinued as well.
      — While a patient receives GVHD prophylaxis, frequent laboratory studies including complete blood count (CBC), renal and hepatic chemistry studies, and cytomegalovirus surveillance are needed.
  - GVHD surveillance involves planned, frequent laboratory studies; diagnostic studies; a review of symptoms; and a physical examination:
    - HSCT recipients are educated about the signs and symptoms of GVHD and taught how to perform self-examinations of the skin and mouth and joint/muscle flexibility. They are taught about the importance of reporting new and worsening symptoms in a timely manner.
    - Common GVHD symptoms encountered by HSCT recipients are detailed in Table 15.2.
    - GVHD diagnosis may involve a review of symptoms, a physical examination, laboratory and radiology studies, biopsies, and an HSCT clinician's expert evaluation of the data.
    - GVHD is described by both histologic grade (if disease is present on tissue biopsy) and clinical stage.
    - Delays in GVHD diagnosis and treatment contribute to poor outcomes.
    - GVHD treatment may be topical or systemic and frequently involves steroid use in high doses for long durations.

TABLE 15.2 Common Graft versus Host Disease Symptoms

Area	Symptoms
Eyes	Constant dryness, irritation or gritty feeling, eye discomfort from air or wind, blurry vision
Throat/esophagus	Difficult and/or painful swallowing
Mouth	Dryness that is new or worsens, discomfort (burning or stinging) when eating certain foods, sores, clear blisters, lacy white or gray skin changes on the inner surfaces
Lips	Tight skin around the lips, lacy white or gray skin growth on the lips, sores
Skin	Rash, redness, spots, sores, or color change; skin feels tight and/or very thick; changes in the feel of skin such as orange peel or firm bumps under the skin, including the skin of the penis or vaginal area
Hair	New hair loss or severe hair thinning on the scalp; hair loss on other areas of the body
Nails	Abnormal growth changes; nails that split or have ridges
Gastrointestinal	Frequent nausea and/or vomiting; loss of appetite; ongoing weight loss; watery diarrhea
Lungs	Ongoing dry cough; shortness of breath at rest or with light activity; wheezing
Joints/muscles	Stiff, tight, or limited movement of the fingers, wrists, elbows, shoulders, hips, knees, or ankles; ongoing muscle aches
Vagina	Dryness, painful intercourse

- o Some GVHD may necessitate combinations of treatments commonly including but not limited to steroids, calcineurin inhibitors (tacrolimus, sirolimus, cyclosporine), extracorporeal photopheresis, and ruxilotinib.
- o GVHD care must be managed by an HSCT expert clinician.

DISEASE SURVEILLANCE AND ENGRAFTMENT

- The HSCT team performs and/or directs disease surveillance and engraftment studies during the most critical period of time after HSCT during which relapse, progression, or graft failure may be anticipated (typically 1–5 years after HSCT):

  - The duration of the critical period is most commonly influenced by the disease for which HSCT is performed, posttransplant medical events, HSCT type, clinical trial requirements as applicable, and GVHD status.
  - The HSCT recipient's community-based oncologist/hematologist should perform disease surveillance when the patient is not able or willing to return to

the HSCT center during the disease-specific time period during which relapse risk is highest. Recommended disease surveillance is outlined in the disease-specific sections of this handbook, or refer to the National Comprehensive Cancer Network.

COMMON LATE/LONG-TERM EFFECTS OF CANCER TREATMENT

- Social, home, and community:

  - Infectious exposure considerations regarding children, pets, travel, and water recreation
  - Poor social reintegration
  - Family role dysfunction
  - Personal relationship stress
  - Loss of employment
  - Financial burden:
    o Past and current medical care
    o Loss of or decreased employment
  - Substance abuse

- Wellness activities/prevention/early detection:

  - Sedentary lifestyle, low physical activity
  - Infection considerations regarding children, pets, travel, and water recreation
  - New cancer risk(s):
    o Hematologic
    o Oral
    o Skin
    o Thyroid
  - Potential need for earlier or more frequent early cancer detection:
    o Annual head-to-toe skin cancer screening examination
    o Annual dental/oral cancer screening
    o Annual CBC
    o Mammogram starting at an earlier age for women who have a history of chest radiation. Begin at age 40 or 8 years after completion of radiation, whichever is earlier
    o Immunizations/vaccinations: HSCT recipients receive a series of four sets of post-HSCT vaccines that begin about 6 months after HSCT and are generally complete by 2 years after HSCT. The initial vaccination plan does not include "live" vaccines. Consideration for live vaccines should be coordinated with the HSCT medical provider because of potential delays in an HSCT recipient's immune reconstitution:
      — A yearly influenza vaccine is recommended for those who are not allergic to the vaccine, people residing in an HSCT recipient's household, and close contacts.

— A pneumococcal vaccination booster is recommended every 5 years after completion of the initial series.

— Patients who have had monoclonal antibodies or other immune therapies that may lead to immune suppression or deficiencies are at risk for reactivation of viral infections such as herpes zoster and hepatitis B and for atypical infections.

— The live shingles vaccine should not be considered unless discussed with an HSCT provider. A nonlive shingles vaccine likely will be available in 2018, and guidelines for use in HSCT survivors are being prepared.

- Emotional/psychiatric:

  - Depression
  - Anxiety
  - Posttraumatic stress disorder
  - Posttraumatic growth
  - Body image disturbance

- Immunologic:

  - Frequent infection or major infections necessitating hospitalization
  - Shingles (herpes zoster)
  - Exacerbations/chronic outbreaks of previous viral infections (hepatitis, genital herpes, skin warts)
  - Poor immune reconstitution:
    o Hypo-gammaglobulinemia
    o Poor T-cell reconstitution (CD4 count)
  - GVHD (see Table 15.2 for types, signs, and symptoms)

- Hematologic:

  - There is a lifelong need for irradiation and leukocyte depletion of red blood cell and platelet transfusion products
  - Poor hematologic reconstitution:
    o Anemia
    o Thrombocytopenia
    o Leukopenia
  - Coagulopathy
  - New blood cancer(s): myelodysplastic syndrome, leukemia
  - Posttransplant lymphoproliferative disease

- Constitutional/endocrine:

  - Fatigue
  - Sleep disorders
  - Obesity
  - Diabetes

- ▪ Thyroid dysfunction:
  - o Hypothyroidism
  - o Hyperthyroidism
  - o Thyroiditis
- ▪ Adrenal insufficiency

- Cognitive:

  - ▪ Short-term memory issues
  - ▪ Concentration/focus issues
  - ▪ Learning/school challenges
  - ▪ Job challenges

- Neurologic:

  - ▪ Peripheral neuropathy
  - ▪ Altered mental status related to medication, disease relapse, or stroke

- Head, ears, eyes, nose, and throat (HEENT):

  - ▪ Dry eye syndrome, ocular GVHD, retinal disease, cataract growth, decreased visual acuity
  - ▪ Hearing loss
  - ▪ Upper respiratory infection
  - ▪ Dry mouth syndrome, accelerated dental caries, oral GVHD, oral cancer
  - ▪ Esophageal stricture/GVHD

- Pulmonary:

  - ▪ Bronchiolitis obliterans syndrome (pulmonary GVHD)
  - ▪ Restrictive lung disorder
  - ▪ Infection

- Cardiac/cardiovascular:

  - ▪ Metabolic syndrome
  - ▪ Early cardiac events:
    - o Myocardial infarction
    - o Stroke
    - o Congestive heart failure
  - ▪ Arrhythmia
  - ▪ Lipid disorder:
    - o Hypercholesterolemia
    - o Hypertriglyceridemia
  - ▪ Clotting disorder:
    - o Deep vein thrombosis
    - o Pulmonary embolis

- Gastrointestinal (GI):

  - Infection:
    - *Clostridium difficile*
    - Viral infection
  - GVHD:
    - Upper GI
    - Lower GI
  - Gastroparesis

- Urinary:

  - Infection
  - Renal insufficiency
  - Renal failure

- Genital:

  - Infection
  - GVHD

- Sexuality/sexual function:

  - Poor libido
  - Inability to reach orgasm
  - Erectile dysfunction

- Fertility:

  - Early menopause
  - Infertility
  - High-risk pregnancy

- Muscles and joints:

  - Infection
  - Deconditioning
  - GVHD

- Skeletal:

  - Low bone density:
    - Osteopenia
    - Osteoporosis
  - Pathologic fracture
  - Avascular necrosis

- Skin:

  - Infection
  - GVHD

- Sun sensitivity
- Skin cancer:
  - Basal cell
  - Squamous cell

REVIEW OF SYSTEMS

- These survivorship-specific guidelines should be used in addition to a typical medical office visit review of systems to enhance assessment of HSCT survivors on an initial and at least annual basis. The review of systems for an HSCT survivor should not be limited to problems. A focus on new or worsening symptoms is useful to help diagnose late effects. A focus on improvements and positive themes during the review of systems also serves as a valuable diagnostic and therapeutic tool. Consider that this person is traveling a road to a personal new normal and may not be able to fully sense his or her own progress during that journey. Do not neglect the opportunity to provide feedback on specific, even modest, improvements, and positive themes that a system review may reveal. The healthcare provider's role includes helping survivors navigate their personal journey.

- Social, home, and community:
  - Marital status change
  - New family members (children, grandchildren)
  - New pets in home
  - Return to work/school:
    - Concerns about return to work/school
    - Change in occupation
  - Leisure, fun, and relaxation activities:
    - Socialization, engagement with friends, family
    - Other community activities (church, volunteer activities, social groups)
    - Recent or planned travel (domestic vs. international)
    - Desire for activities/socialization (but feel they cannot participate because of limitations)
  - Relationship(s) with spouse/significant other(s), friends, family:
    - Relationship stress
  - Money worries:
    - Personal/family finances, trouble meeting basic bill payments such as utilities, rent, or mortgage
    - Missing recommended medical follow-ups because of money problems
    - Medical insurance loss/changes
  - Substance use:
    - Tobacco products
    - Inhaled e-cigarettes
    - Alcohol
    - Marijuana products
    - Other nonprescribed drug product

- Wellness activities/prevention/early detection:

  - Current planned exercise: Type, typical duration of activity, how often
  - Current use of sun protection (what and when)
  - Immunizations (what and when)
  - Date of most recent:
    - Mammogram
    - Pelvic examination
    - Prostate examination/prostate-specific antigen test
    - Colonoscopy
    - Head-to-toe skin examination
    - Eye examination
    - Dental examination
    - Bone density study

- Emotional/psychiatric:

  - Depression
  - Anxiety
  - Sadness
  - Worry
  - Stress
  - Body image disturbance

- Immunologic:

  - Recent infections/frequency of infections
  - Pneumonia
  - Upper respiratory
  - Shingles
  - Skin infections
  - GI infections
  - GVHD:
    - Current use of GVHD prevention medication: none, tacrolimus, sirolimus, or cyclosporine
    - Site of current GVHD: None, eyes, mouth, skin, GI tract, liver, joints/muscles, other
    - Current symptoms: none or GHVD symptoms as listed in Table 15.2
    - Provider managing GVHD
    - Current treatments for GVHD:
      — Medications:
        a. Tacrolimus, sirolimus, cyclosporine, mycophenolate mofetil, ruxolitinib for various systemic forms of GVHD
        b. Methylprednisolone or prednisone for skin, GI, liver, joints/muscles, budesonide (for upper GI)
        c. Topical steroid (hydrocortisone, triamcinolone for skin)
        d. Cyclosporine eye drops, autologous serum tears for eye(s)
        e. Dexamethasone oral rinse for mouth

— Procedures:
  a. Punctual cautery for eyes
  b. Punctual plugs for eyes
  c. Extracorporeal photopheresis of skin, liver
  d. Physical therapy for joints/muscles, fasciitis
— Devices:
  a. Specialized contact lenses

- Hematologic
  - Adenopathy
  - Easy bleeding and bruising
  - Current use of hematologic growth factor(s) (filgrastim, erythropoietin, eltrombopag)

- Constitutional:
  - Activity level
  - Typical day, napping
  - Energy
  - Fatigue
  - Sleep:
    o Chronic use of sleep medication
    o Insomnia
    o Waking and not being able to go back to sleep
    o Frequent multiple sleep disturbances
  - Appetite:
    o Poor appetite
    o No sensation of being hungry
    o Taste changes make food unappealing
    o Early satiety
    o Ravenous appetite
  - Unplanned weight change
  - Unusual thirst

- Cognitive:
  - Short-term memory deficit
  - Trouble concentrating
  - Trouble multitasking
  - Word finding
  - Difficulty learning new things

- Neurologic:
  - Numbness, tingling, or discomfort in fingers, hands, toes, or feet
  - Balance issue or falls attributable to neuropathy
  - Poor sleep attributable to neuropathy
  - Difficulty pulling up zippers, buttoning clothing, picking up coins

- Cold sensitivity of hands/feet
- Light-headed/dizzy
- Fainting
- Fall(s)

- HEENT:

  - Eyes: Dry eyes, gritty feeling in eyes, air or wind irritates eyes, changes in vision
  - Ears: New or worsening hearing loss
  - Nose: Congestion, rhinorrhea, postnasal drip
  - Mouth: Dryness, dental sensitivity, breaking teeth, oral membrane sensitivity/pain, mouth sores or lesions, mucoceles, tissue pigmentation change, new lumps or bumps, growths
  - Lips: Pigmentation change, sores, tightness of lips
  - Neck: Lumps or swollen lymph nodes
  - Throat: Difficulty swallowing

- Pulmonary:

  - Cough
  - Wheezing
  - Shortness of breath with very low activity or at rest:
    - Use of oxygen
    - Use of inhaler(s)
  - Apnea (sleep related):
    - Use of continuous positive airway pressure therapy

- Cardiac/cardiovascular:

  - Chest discomfort with activity
  - Rapid heart rate
  - Palpitations
  - Swelling of face, hands, arms, and feet/legs
  - Leg/calf pain when walking
  - Hip/knee/shoulder pain when weight bearing

- GI:

  - Nausea: Assess frequency, medication use
  - Vomiting: Assess frequency, medication use, blood in emesis
  - Diarrhea: Assess frequency, consistency, urgency, volume, blood in stool
  - Constipation
  - Abdominal pain, cramping
  - Frequent indigestion/reflux symptoms

- Urinary:

  - Urgency, difficulty controlling urine
  - Frequency

- Dribbling or low force of urine stream
- Low urine volume
- Unusually large urine volume
- Pain/discomfort with urination
- Blood in urine

- Genital:

  - Sores/lesions or skin changes on penis, vagina, or rectal areas
  - Penile/vaginal pain
  - Unusual/unexpected vaginal bleeding

- Sexuality/sexual function:

  - Low sexual desire/low libido
  - Pain with sexual activity
  - Loss of pleasure with sexual activity
  - Inability to have orgasm
  - Erectile dysfunction
  - Feeling less attractive to partner
  - Partner communication challenges

- Fertility:

  - Current use of birth control
  - Return or cessation of menstrual periods
  - Hot flashes
  - Family building:
    - o Desire/future plans
    - o Prechemotherapy sperm or egg cryopreservation
      - — Financial ability to maintain storage
    - o Fertility testing since HSCT
    - o Conception since transplant
    - o Live birth/miscarriage since transplant

- Muscles and joints:

  - Muscle aches
  - Muscle cramps or spasms
  - Change in range of motion attributable to muscle tightness or pain:
    - o Frequency, site(s), limitation(s)
    - o Joint pain/aches
  - Change in range of motion attributable to joint tightness or pain
    - o Frequency, site(s), limitation(s)

- Skeletal:

  - Bone pain (weight bearing or at rest)

- Skin:

  - Color/pigment changes
  - Rash
  - Sensation changes such as heat or sun sensitivity, numbness, and pain
  - New moles or skin lesions, changes in moles, mole or skin lesion bleeding
  - Tightening or thickening of skin
  - Unusual nail characteristics
  - Unusual hair growth characteristics/hair loss

PHYSICAL EXAMINATION

In addition to performing a typical medical visit physical examination, take this opportunity to enhance your HSCT survivor assessment.

- Constitutional:

  - Personal hygiene
  - Alertness
  - Weight, body mass index
  - Body habitus:
    o Obesity
    o Cachexia

- Emotional/psychiatric:

  - Eye contact
  - Affect
  - Responses to questions, interaction, engagement
  - Orderliness of thought processes

- Neurologic:

  - Gait
  - Foot placement during walking
  - Ability to pick up coins off of a flat surface

- HEENT:

  - Eyes: Red and irritable appearance, excessive tearing, frequent use of moisturizing eye drops during examination
  - Nose: Congestion, rhinorrhea
  - Mouth: Dryness, membrane color, lesions, mucoceles, lichenoid changes on membranes, breaking teeth, pigmentation change of tissues, growths
  - Oral pharynx: Postnasal drip
  - Lips: Pigmentation change, sores, tightness
  - Neck: Cervical, submandibular, periauricular, or supraclavicular adenopathy; thyroid size; tenderness; nodules

- Pulmonary:
  - Cough
  - Wheezing
  - Shortness of breath
  - Use of oxygen

- Cardiac/cardiovascular:
  - Heart rate
  - Arrhythmia
  - Murmur
  - Edema (face, hands, arms, feet/legs)

- Abdominal:
  - Bloating, ascites, bowel sounds, pain on palpation

- Genital:
  - Inguinal adenopathy
  - Scrotal edema, masses
  - Sores/lesions or skin changes of the penis, vaginal, or rectal areas
  - Pelvic examination: Atrophy of vaginal tissues, dryness, stricture of vaginal vault, agglutination of vaginal tissues

- Muscles and joints:
  - Range-of-motion examination of shoulders, elbows, wrists, fingers, hips, knees, and ankles

- Skin:
  - Color/pigment changes
  - Rash
  - New moles or skin lesions, mole changes, mole or skin lesion bleeding
  - Tightening or thickening of skin, especially in axillary, thoracic, inner thigh, and ankles/lower calves
  - Axillary adenopathy
  - Unusual nail characteristics
  - Unusual hair growth characteristics/hair loss
  - Other changes per the National Comprehensive Cancer Network's disease surveillance guidelines

RECOMMENDED LABORATORY TESTS

These tests are specific to common late effects experienced by HSCT survivors. Survivors with ongoing immunosuppressive medication requirements may need more frequent monitoring, and the HSCT team typically will provide that direction.

- CBC with differential and platelet count, at least annually, to check for anemia, abnormal platelet count, or leukocyte population changes
- Chemistry profile, at least annually, to monitor for vital organ function including liver and kidney; monitoring of metabolic parameters (glucose, albumin, total protein, etc.); diabetes and chronic kidney disease are common late effects
- Immunoglobulin level findings (IgG, IgA, IgM), which may elucidate the cause of recurrent infections, help to monitor recovery of B-cell function, and reveal monoclonal gammopathy
- Thyroid-stimulating hormone and T4 lab tests annually to monitor for hypothyroidism (most common), hyperthyroidism, or thyroiditis
- Vitamin D level annually to monitor for deficiency that may impact bone health (vitamin D supplementation likely will be needed)
- Lipid profile to monitor for high low-density lipoprotein (LDL) and low high-density lipoprotein (HDL) levels, which may impact cardiac health; strongly recommend dietary, physical activity, and weight and statin management

RECOMMENDED RADIOLOGIC/DIAGNOSTIC PROCEDURES

- Chest x-ray to assess for symptoms of lower respiratory infection; pneumonia is a common late infection for HSCT recipients
- Pulmonary function test to assess for new or chronic respiratory symptoms, especially when they occur weeks to months after recovery of respiratory infection, which may indicate pulmonary GVHD or bronchiolitis obliterans syndrome in allogeneic HSCT survivors. Check for a decline in the first forced expiratory volume of 10% or more. Refer to a pulmonologist or HSCT medical team
- A baseline bone mineral density study is recommended during the first year after HSCT for men and women of all ages because of the common late effects of osteopenia and osteoporosis. Ongoing monitoring is needed every 2 to 3 years if history includes menopause, ongoing steroid use, osteopenia, and osteoporosis. Treat osteoporosis and consider referral to an endocrinologist or community bone health specialist
- Electrocardiogram to assess for history and ongoing monitoring for new rhythm changes. Cardiac arrhythmias may manifest years after receiving chemotherapy or radiation therapy
- For new-onset murmur or cardiac insufficiency symptoms, consider an echocardiogram. There is controversy regarding the frequency of routine echocardiograms for patients who have received anthracyclines and/or mediastinal radiation
- Doppler ultrasound of carotids: Consider if the HSCT survivor has a carotid bruit upon examination, a history of neck node radiation attributable to risk for carotid stenosis, or has been taking long-term calcineurin inhibitor therapy to address risk for atherosclerosis
- Refer to the MD Anderson clinical practice algorithms, Pregnancy Screening, Fertility Preservation to Cancer Treatment, and Fertility Sparing Treatment (available at www.mdanderson.org)
- Fertility preservation should be recommended for patients of childbearing age
- Refer to fertility clinics and/or online fertility resources

RISK REDUCTION/EARLY DETECTION

- Breast screening
  Eight to 10 years posttreatment (if treated with radiation to the chest or axilla) or at age 40, whichever comes first; continue annual screening

- Skin screening
  Because of immunosuppressive therapy history and potential past radiation and skin GVHD, a head-to-toe skin examination is recommended at least yearly

- Vaccinations
  HSCT recipients receive a series of four sets of post-HSCT vaccines that begin about 6 months after HSCT and are generally complete by 2 years after HSCT. The initial vaccination plan does not include "live" vaccines. Consideration for live vaccines should be coordinated with the HSCT medical provider because of potential delays in an HSCT recipient's immune reconstitution:

  - A yearly influenza vaccine is recommended for those who are not allergic to the vaccine and for people residing in an HSCT recipient's household and close contacts.
  - A pneumococcal vaccination booster is recommended every 5 years after completion of the initial series.
  - Patients who have had monoclonal antibodies or other immune therapies that may lead to immune suppression or deficiencies are at risk for reactivation of viral infections such as herpes zoster and hepatitis B as well as atypical infections.
  - The shingles vaccine is live and should not be considered unless discussed with an HSCT provider.

PSYCHOSOCIAL HEALTH AND FUNCTIONING

Because of the potential complexity and cascading nature of these issues, an in-depth assessment is warranted.

- Fatigue: Ongoing fatigue can be a factor in an HSCT survivor's overall quality of life. Assess fatigue scores and provide information about energy conservation, sleep hygiene, and physical activity to improve this score
- Relationship issues: Evolving roles within a family and survivor's close social circle during cancer treatment and recovery may take time to normalize. HSCT survivors, family members, and friends may move through this adjustment period differently and have disparate expectations. Relationship stress is a common late effect. Inquire about family and social relationships. Promote communication between parents/spouse/partners/siblings. Encourage participation in and provide information about psychosocial support and behavioral services, support groups, social and recreational programs, and couples or family counseling services. Consider a referral to social services

- Social isolation: Because of long periods of treatment, recovery, and immunodeficiency, HSCT survivors may be delayed in reengaging with friends and coworkers. Inquire about the ways in which survivors spend their free time, what they choose to do for recreation, and if they are reengaging in social relationships. Note that adolescent and young adult survivors may be particularly vulnerable to isolation. Encourage social reintegration and consider referral to age-appropriate support or social groups
- Body image: HSCT survivors may experience weight changes attributable to treatments and long-term medication use, muscle loss, steroid-related facial changes, and long-term skin pigmentation or hair growth pattern changes. Ask HSCT survivors if they are experiencing discomfort with body changes
- Access to primary healthcare (refer to primary care providers)
- Employment and return-to-school stressors:

  - Employment issues:
    - o Cancer treatment effects such as chronic fatigue, pain, neuropathy, and cognitive and sensory impairments; ongoing immunodeficiency; and potential toxic exposures can interfere with a survivor's ability to perform certain types of work. Advise patients about possible challenges they may face as they go back to work or school, such as the need to decrease work load or hours, transition from full-time to part-time, or change jobs.
    - o Encourage HSCT survivors to inquire about accommodations for which they may be eligible at their place of employment.
    - o Consider a social work referral for information on available government assistance.
    - o Consider a referral to vocational rehabilitation or counseling.
    - o Consider a referral to school counselors and school advocates for adolescent and young adults who may need to reconcile class withdrawals and transcript consequences attributable to cancer treatment. There also may be financial assistance for secondary education for cancer survivors.
    - o Assist patients with Family and Medical Leave Act applications and provide supporting letters for job restrictions/limitations.

- Financial stressors:

  - Financial burden resulting from treatment cost can persist throughout the survivorship period. Studies show that financial burden is associated with poor patient outcomes and increased mortality. Older HSCT survivors may be particularly vulnerable to financial distress because of limited income, inability to work, and the need for unplanned early retirement:
    - o Assess for financial issues.
    - o Provide lists of local or national services or organizations such as the Lymphoma and Leukemia Society.
    - o Link qualified survivors to Medicaid, Social Security, and/or disability insurance/transportation programs.
  - Consider a social work or case manager referral.

RESOURCES

Caring for HSCT survivors can be complex, so consider using community and national resources. Consult with experienced oncology professionals and stem cell transplantation teams. Survivor-oriented online resources for HSCT survivors also may be helpful for primary care providers. Three of these valuable resources are the following:

- National Marrow Donor Program's Be the Match at www.bethematch.org, which offers a section for healthcare providers and patients that addresses the continuum of care pretransplant through long-term survival
- Bone and Marrow Transplant Information Network at www.BMTinfonet.org for patient newsletters and online free webcasts that address many posttransplant survivorship issues
- National Bone Marrow Transplant Link at www.nbmtlink.org, which features articles, videos, and books of interest to HSCT survivors

CLINICAL VIGNETTE

RHS comes to your family practice office to establish herself as a new patient. She is a 28-year-old female with a history of B-cell precursor acute lymphoblastic leukemia who has received chemotherapy and bone marrow transplant (referred to as a HSCT in this chapter). She is now 4 years after HSCT, in continuous complete remission. She has been working full time as an early childhood teacher, teaching children ages 3 and 4 for about 18 months. She provides a verbal history and gives a treatment summary prepared by her treating HSCT team at time of initial discharge from the HSCT center (about day 100 after transplant [see the following paragraphs]). She was given a recommended long-term follow-up plan, but did not bring it with her.

Brief History

RHS was diagnosed with B-cell precursor acute lymphoblastic leukemia at age 17, in her senior year of high school. She received treatment with induction, consolidation, and maintenance chemotherapy, as well as chemotherapy into the cerebrospinal fluid as central nervous system prophylaxis. Her treatment took about 11 months to complete. She achieved a complete remission after her first cycle of chemotherapy and remained in complete remission. She was able to complete high school during her year of treatment.

She then earned a college degree in early childhood education. As she was about to enter the work force as an early childhood teacher at age 23, she relapsed with acute lymphoblastic leukemia. She received more chemotherapy, including a clinical trial drug, and after four cycles still had residual leukemia. She then received two cycles of immunotherapy drugs, achieving a complete remission.

Her B-cell precursor leukemia proved to be aggressive and a high risk for recurrence, so she received further therapy to increase her chance for cure, in the form of HSCT. A matched unrelated female donor was found through the international bone marrow transplant registry. To prepare her body to receive the donor marrow, she received a conditioning regimen of total body irradiation (TBI), a total of 12 Gray given in four fractions, and chemotherapy, etoposide, followed by the donor marrow infusion.

In her first year posttransplant, she developed limited GVHD requiring treatment with steroid creams. It resolved quickly. She also developed GVHD of the upper gastrointestinal tract causing persistent nausea, and weight loss. It was treated with budesonide for about 3 months. She has been off of all immunosuppression for more than 2 years.

Cancer Treatment Summary Provided on 04/19/2014	
General Information	
Patient Name	RHS
Patient ID	000000
Date of Birth	00/00/0000
Age	24 y.o.
Sex	Female
Allergies	Penicillins
Providers	
Survivorship Care Provider	Karen Stolar FNP-BC
Stem Cell Transplant Physician	Mary Smith, MD

Transfusion: All blood products infused must be IRRADIATED and leukodepleted (white cell filtered, leuko poor).
Background Information

Past Medical History	
Diagnosis	Date
Acute lymphoblastic leukemia	

(continued)

Cancer Treatment Summary (*continued*)	
Cancer Diagnosis Information	
Cancer Diagnosis	Acute lymphoid leukemia, B-cell precursor
Date of Diagnosis	10/2008
History of Central Nervous System Involvement	No
Mutations/Cytogenetics at Diagnosis	No record found from outside hospital.
Other Disease Characteristics at Diagnosis	Bone marrow showing 66% blasts consistent with B-cell lymphoblastic leukemia/lymphoma.
Pretransplant Chronologic Treatment History	
Date	Treatment
8/2008–3/2009	Augmented Berlin-Frankfurt-Münster induction and four consolidation cycles (Daunorubicin, Vincristine, Prednisone, PEG-asparaginase Intrathecal cytarabine, Intrathecal methotrexate, Cyclophosphamide, 6-Mercaptopurine) Entered complete remission with induction cycle.
4/8/2009–8/26/2009	BFM maintenance × six cycles
9/2014	**Relapse.**
9/2013–10/2013	Protocol: XXXX, Mini hyper CVAD (cyclophosphamide, vincristine, doxorubicin, dexamethasone alternating with cytarabine, methotrexate) + CMC- 544 + rituximab × 2 cycles, + Intrathecal chemotherapy. Result: persistent minimal residual disease
11/2013–12/2013	Blinatumumab, two cycles
Stem Cell Transplant History	
Disease Status at Transplant	No minimal residual disease.
Date of Transplant	1/11/2014
Donor Type	Matched Unrelated

Cancer Treatment Summary (*continued*)			
Stem Cell Source	Marrow		
Recipient Original Blood Type	B Positive		
Recipient Pretrans-plant CMV Status	CMV Negative		
	Donor Blood Type	CMV Status	Sex
#1	B Positive	CMV Negative	Female
Conditioning Regimen	Total body irradiation (12 Gy total in four fractions), etopo-side, ATG	Standard of Care	
Posttransplant Mainte-nance Drug	None		
Graft versus Host Disease (GVHD) Prevention	Tacrolimus and methotrexate		

Graft versus Host Disease				
Site(s)		Treatment(s)	Current status	
Skin		Topical steroids	Resolved	
Gastrointestinal		Budesonide	Resolved	
Other Cell Therapies History	No			
Engraftment Study 3/11/2014	T cells	100 %	Myeloid cells	100 %	are of donor origin
Disease Status	3/11/2014 Specimen Type: Bone Marrow. Interpreta-tion: Negative for minimal residual precursor-B acute lymphoblastic leukemia			

For questions regarding this patient's care please notify appropriate provider listed earlier.

Facility Affiliation	MD Anderson Cancer Center

(*continued*)

Cancer Treatment Summary (*continued*)	
Clinic Phone	xxx-xxx-xxxx Hours: Monday–Friday, 7:30 a.m.–5 p.m.
Fax Number	xxx-xxx-xxxx
After Hours Page Operator	xxx-xxx-xxxx

Note: The data on this plan are fictional.

1. Because this visit is during influenza season, you ask her about
   A. Number and severity of colds or flu in the last few months
   B. Current upper respiratory symptoms
   C. Receipt of influenza vaccine this flu season
   D. All of the above
   E. Only A and B

2. RHS reports that she is feeling tired lately, her skin is very dry, and her hair seems to be thinning the last month or so. The most appropriate laboratory study(ies) you would order
   A. CBC
   B. Thyroid panel
   C. Lipid panel
   D. A and B
   E. All of the above

3. You notice that RHS is taking vitamin D, calcium, and a bisphosphonate. She tells you she has been diagnosed with osteoporosis, and she gives you a copy of her last bone density study performed about 6 months ago. You will
   A. Advise weight bearing exercise
   B. Order a bone density study in about 6 months
   C. Remind patient to let her dentist know she is taking a bisphosphonate, especially if she needs dental work
   D. Check a vitamin D, 25OH level
   E. All of the above

4. RHS tells you she is getting married in a few months and will be honeymooning in Hawaii. This information gives you a good opening to discuss
   A. Risks of sun exposure and eye and skin protection
   B. Sexuality, physical symptoms, or other concerns
   C. Family building plans and fertility
   D. All of the above
   E. None of the above

TIP

A cancer survivor, especially HSCT survivor, has an extensive and likely complicated history of treatment over many years. Do not let the medical information overwhelm you. Although it is all important for the survivor's long-term plan to provide appropriate care and monitoring, the first visit is an opportunity to get to know the survivor and his or her personal cancer journey. Address immediate concerns and develop the long-term follow-up plan over time with the survivor.

Answers

1. D
Number and severity of respiratory infections can give a hint to the patient's current immune status. Some HSCT survivors' immune function recovery can be delayed or impacted by environmental factors. A HSCT survivor is vulnerable to pneumonia lifelong, should receive a seasonal NON-LIVE influenza vaccine yearly, as well as pneumococcal vaccine series post-transplant and then every 5 years. Address upper respiratory symptoms and associated symptoms, determine if viral testing, strep testing, or chest x-ray is needed.

2. D
Thyroid dysfunction is a frequent late effect of cancer treatment, especially in survivors who have received the high doses of chemotherapy required for HSCT. Total body irradiation is a risk factor for thyroid dysfunction. A thyroid panel is indicated. The risk for relapse in any leukemia survivor is high. Some viral illnesses may impact blood counts, so a complete blood count is also indicated. Although a lipid panel is a recommended long-term follow-up test for HSCT survivors who may be at risk for cardiac late effects, it is not the most appropriate in this scenario.

3. E
Chemotherapy, especially high dose chemotherapy, immunosuppressive medications such as tacrolimus and steroids, and early menopause make this 28-year-old woman vulnerable to the late effect of loss of bone density. Indeed she has osteoporosis and is on treatment with calcium, vitamin D, and bisphosphonates. You should advise weight bearing exercise, check vitamin D 25, OH to be sure her vitamin D level is sufficient, do a follow-up bone density study yearly while on treatment (to be sure the treatment is showing some improvement in bone density and to determine length of treatment). If the treatment is not effective or you are unsure about stopping

treatment, strongly consider a referral to an endocrinologist for evaluation and treatment advice. Bisphosphonate therapy is known to increase risk for osteonecrosis of the mandible or maxilla and the dentist must always be aware that the patient is on a bisphosphonate when considering dental treatment.

4. D

Chemotherapy and/or radiation therapy increases risk for skin cancers, so solar protection is advised. Recommend sunscreen that provides SPF 30 or higher, frequent reapplication while in the sun and after being in the water, as well as sun protective clothing and a hat. Remind RHS that even a cloudy day can allow solar radiation exposure and precautions are needed. The delicate skin around the eyes also needs protection, as well as the eyes. Chemotherapy and/or radiation therapy also increases the risk of cataract development. Ultraviolet (UV) eye protection may provide some delay of that risk. Recommend use of UV protective sunglasses. GVHD of the skin may be activated by unprotected sun exposure in allogeneic HSCT recipients, so the above protections are recommended. A rash that develops within a week or 2 of sun exposure could be GVHD of the skin. Stem cell tranplantation team or dermatologist evaluation may be necessary, especially if it is spreading or is not improving in a day or 2.

Sexuality issues are common in HSCT survivors. Women report poor libido, vaginal dryness, dyspareunia, and inability to reach orgasm. Women also report body image disturbances that may impact their sexuality. Low female hormone status of early menopause and GVHD of the vaginal tissues can also cause dyspareunia, vaginal dryness, and vaginal stenosis. Referral to a gynecologist, especially one who may serve a HSCT center, can be a valuable resource for this patient if she is experiencing any of these issues. Ask directly about these symptoms, as survivors may be reluctant to report a symptom or bring up some of these issues.

Early menopause and infertility after as much chemotherapy as this patient has had is likely. Ask about fertility testing and/or prior oocyte preservation. Referral to OB/GYN or fertility specialist for fertility determination may be something a young woman may want to pursue, particularly if she has not done it before this time period. Ask the HSCT survivor if family building is something she has discussed with her fiancé and may have concerns about. If adoption or surrogacy is something she may want to explore, there are community resources out there to access. If social services do not have the answers for you, a fertility specialist office may have local resources they can share with you.

RECOMMENDED READINGS

Andrykowski MA, Bishop MM, Hahn EA, et al. Long-term health-related quality of life, growth, and spiritual well-being after hematopoietic stem-cell transplantation. *J Clin Oncol*. 2005;23(3):599–608. doi:10.1200/JCO.2005.03.189

Bishop MM, Wingard JR. Thriving after hematopoietic stem cell transplant: a focus on positive changes in quality of life. *Expert Rev Pharmacoecon Outcomes Res*. 2004;4(1):111–123. doi:10.1586/14737167.4.1.111

Bjorklund A, Aschan J, Labopin M, et al. Risk factors for fatal infectious complications developing late after allogeneic stem cell transplantation. *Bone Marrow Transplant*. 2007;40(11):1055–1062. doi:10.1038/sj.bmt.1705856

Carter A, Robison L, Francisco L, et al. Prevalence of conception and pregnancy outcomes after hematopoietic cell transplantation: report from the Bone Marrow Transplant Survivor Study. *Bone Marrow Transplant*. 2006;37(11):1023–1029. doi:10.1038/sj.bmt.1705364

Chang G, Orav J, Mcnamara TK, et al. Psychosocial function after hematopoietic stem cell transplantation. *Psychosomatics*. 2005;46(1):34–40.

Denlinger CS, Ligibel JA, Are M, et al. NCCN guidelines insights: survivorship, version 1.2016. *J Natl Compr Canc Netw*. 2016;14(6):715–724. doi:10.6004/jnccn.2016.0073

Dorland HF, Abma FI, Roelen CAM, et al. The cognitive symptom checklist-work in cancer patients is related with work functioning, fatigue and depressive symptoms: a validation study. *J Cancer Surviv*. 2016;10(3):545–552. doi:10.1007/s11764-015-0500-9

Dudek AZ, Mahaseth H. Hematopoietic stem cell transplant–related airflow obstruction. *Curr Opin Oncol*. 2006;18(2):115–119. doi:10.1097/01.cco.0000208782.61452.08

El-Jawahri A, Chen YB, Brazauskas R, et al. Impact of pre-transplant depression on outcomes of allogeneic and autologous hematopoietic stem cell transplantation. *Cancer*. 2017;123(10):1828–1838. doi:10.1002/cncr.30546

Friedberg JW. Secondary malignancies after therapy of indolent non-Hodgkin's lymphoma. *Haematologica*. 2008;93(3):336–338. doi:10.3324/haematol.12585

Grundy SM. Cardiovascular and metabolic risk factors: how can we improve outcomes in the high-risk patient? *Am J Med*. 2007;120(9):S3–S8. doi:10.1016/j.amjmed.2007.06.005

Jacobs SR, Small BJ, Booth-Jones M, et al. Changes in cognitive functioning in the year after hematopoietic stem cell transplantation. *Cancer*. 2007;110(7):1560–1567. doi:10.1002/cncr.22962

Jones S, Ziebell R, Walker R, et al. Association of worry about cancer to benefit finding and functioning in long-term cancer survivors. *Support Care Cancer*. 2017;25(5):1417–1422. doi:10.1007/s00520-016-3537-z

Lee SJ, Loberiza F, Antin J, et al. Routine screening for psychosocial distress following hematopoietic stem cell transplantation. *Bone Marrow Transplant*. 2005;35(1):77–83. doi:10.1038/sj.bmt.1704709

Majhail NS. Old and new cancers after hematopoietic-cell transplantation. *ASH Education Program Book*. 2008;2008(1):142–149. doi:10.1182/asheducation-2008.1.142

Majhail NS, Brazauskas R, Rizzo JD, et al. Secondary solid cancers after allogeneic hematopoietic cell transplantation using busulfan-cyclophosphamide conditioning. *Blood*. 2011;117(1):316–322. doi:10.1182/blood-2010-07-294629

Majhail NS, Rizzo JD, Lee SJ, et al. Recommended screening and preventive practices for long-term survivors after hematopoietic cell transplantation. *Hematol Oncol Stem Cell Ther*. 2012;5(1):1–30. doi:10.5144/1658-3876.2012.1

Massenkeil G, Fiene C, Rosen O, et al. Loss of bone mass and vitamin D deficiency after hematopoietic stem cell transplantation: standard prophylactic measures fail to prevent osteoporosis. *Leukemia.* 2001;15(11):1701.

Melisko ME, Narus JB. Sexual function in cancer survivors: updates to the NCCN guidelines for survivorship. *J Natl Compr Canc Netw.* 2016;14(suppl 5):685–689. doi:10.6004/jnccn.2016.0193

Mohty M, Apperley JF. Long-term physiological side effects after allogeneic bone marrow transplantation. *ASH Educ Program Book.* 2010;2010(1):229–236. doi:10.1182/asheducation-2010.1.229

Mosher CE, Redd WH, Rini CM, et al. Physical, psychological, and social sequelae following hematopoietic stem cell transplantation: a review of the literature. *Psycho-Oncology.* 2009;18(2):113–127. doi:10.1002/pon.1399

Naughton MJ, Weaver KE. Physical and mental health among cancer survivors considerations for long-term care and quality of life. *N C Med J.* 2014;75(4):283–286. doi:10.18043/ncm.75.4.283

Nekhlyudov L, Walker R, Ziebell R, et al. Cancer survivors' experiences with insurance, finances, and employment: results from a multisite study. *J Cancer Surviv.* 2016;10(6):1104–1111. doi:10.1007/s11764-016-0554-3

Pandya CM, Soubani AO. Bronchiolitis obliterans following hematopoietic stem cell transplantation: a clinical update. *Clin Transplant.* 2010;24(3):291–306. doi:10.1111/j.1399-0012.2009.01122.x

Patriarca F, Poletti V, Costabel U, et al. Clinical presentation, outcome and risk factors of late-onset non-infectious pulmonary complications after allogeneic stem cell transplantation. *Curr Stem Cell Res Ther.* 2009;4(2):161–167. doi:10.2174/157488809788167436

Polomano RC, Farrar JT. Pain and neuropathy in cancer survivors. Surgery, radiation, and chemotherapy can cause pain; research could improve its detection and treatment. *Am J Nurs.* 2006;106(Suppl 3):39–47.

Poppelreuter M, Weis J, Mumm A, et al. Rehabilitation of therapy-related cognitive deficits in patients after hematopoietic stem cell transplantation. *Bone Marrow Transplant.* 2008;41(1):79–90. doi:10.1038/sj.bmt.1705884

Rizzo JD, Curtis RE, Socié G, et al. Solid cancers after allogeneic hematopoietic cell transplantation. *Blood.* 2009;113(5):1175–1183. doi: 10.1182/blood-2008-05-158782

Rizzo JD, Wingard JR, Tichelli A, et al. Recommended screening and preventive practices for long-term survivors after hematopoietic cell transplantation: joint recommendations of the European group for blood and marrow transplantation, the center for international blood and marrow transplant research, and the American society of blood and marrow transplantation. *Biol Blood Marrow Transplant.* 2006;12(2):138–151. doi:10.1016/j.bbmt.2011.12.519

Robin M, Porcher R, Araujo RDC, et al. Risk factors for late infections after allogeneic hematopoietic stem cell transplantation from a matched related donor. *Biol Blood Marrow Transplant.* 2007;13(11):1304–1312. doi:10.1016/j.bbmt.2007.07.007

Roziakova L, Mladosievicova B. Endocrine late effects after hematopoietic stem cell transplantation. *Oncology Research Featuring Preclinical and Clinical Cancer Therapeutics.* 2009;18(11-12):607–615.

Sacchi S, Marcheselli L, Bari A, et al. Secondary malignancies after treatment for indolent non-Hodgkin's lymphoma: a 16-year follow-up study. *Haematologica.* 2008;93(3):398–404. doi:10.3324/haematol.12120

Savani BN, Koklanaris EK, Le Q, et al. Prolonged chronic graft-versus-host disease is a risk factor for thyroid failure in long-term survivors after matched sibling donor stem cell transplantation for hematologic malignancies. *Biol Blood Marrow Transplant*. 2009;15(3):377–381. doi:10.1016/j.bbmt.2008.11.032

Schulmeister L, Quiett K, Mayer K. Quality of life, quality of care, and patient satisfaction: perceptions of patients undergoing outpatient autologous stem cell transplantation. *Oncology Nursing Forum*. 2005;32(1):57–67. doi:10.1188/05.ONF.57-67

Schwartz JL, Kopecky KJ, Mathes RW, et al. Basal cell skin cancer after total-body irradiation and hematopoietic cell transplantation. *Radiat Res*. 2009;171(2):155–163. doi:10.1667/RR1469.1

Shanklin V, Snowden J, Greenfield D. Late treatment effects following bone marrow transplant: efficacy of implementing international guidelines. *Eur J Cancer Care*. 2018; Mar27(2):e12623. doi:10.1111.ecc.12623

Socié G, Salooja N, Cohen A, et al. Nonmalignant late effects after allogeneic stem cell transplantation. *Blood*. 2003;101(9):3373–3385. doi:10.1182/blood-2002-07-2231

Socie G, Tichelli A. Long-term care after stem-cell transplantation. *Hematol J*. 2004;5:S39. doi:10.1038/sj.thj.6200420

Stergiou-Kita M, Pritlove C, Holness DL, et al. Am I ready to return to work? Assisting cancer survivors to determine work readiness. *J Cancer Surviv*. 2016;10(4):699–710. doi:10.1007/s11764-016-0516-9

Stolar K, Alousi A, Neumann J, et al. Hematologic cancer survivorship management: transplantation. In: Foxhall LE, Rodriguez MA, eds. *Advances in Cancer Survivorship Management*. New York, NY: Springer; 2015:167–186.

Syrjala KL, Kurland BF, Abrams JR, et al. Sexual function changes during the 5 years after high-dose treatment and hematopoietic cell transplantation for malignancy, with case-matched controls at 5 years. *Blood*. 2008;111(3):989–996. doi:10.1182/blood-2007-06-096594

Syrjala KL, Langer SL, Abrams JR, et al. Late effects of hematopoietic cell transplantation among 10-year adult survivors compared with case-matched controls. *J Clin Oncol*. 2005;23(27):6596–6606. doi:10.1200/JCO.2005.12.674

Syrjala KL, Yi JC, Artherholt SB, et al. Measuring musculoskeletal symptoms in cancer survivors who receive hematopoietic cell transplantation. *J Cancer Surviv*. 2010;4(3):225–235. doi:10.1007/s11764-010-0126-x

Tichelli A, Bucher C, Rovó A, et al. Premature cardiovascular disease after allogeneic hematopoietic stem-cell transplantation. *Blood*. 2007;110(9):3463–3471. doi:10.1182/blood-2006-10-054080

Tichelli A, Rovó A, Passweg J, et al. Late complications after hematopoietic stem cell transplantation. *Expert Rev Hematol*. 2009;2(5):583–601. doi:10.1586/ehm.09.48

Tierney DK. Sexuality following hematopoietic cell transplantation. *Clin J Oncol Nurs*. 2004;8(1):43–47.

Tomblyn M, Chiller T, Einsele H, et al. Guidelines for preventing infectious complications among hematopoietic cell transplantation recipients: a global perspective. *Biol Blood Marrow Transplant*. 2009;15(10):1143–1238. doi:10.1016/j.bbmt.2009.06.019

Walker E, Martins A, Aldiss S, et al. Psychosocial interventions for adolescents and young adults diagnosed with cancer during adolescence: a critical review. *J Adolesc Young Adult Oncol*. 2016;5(4):310–321. doi:10.1089/jayao.2016.0025

Worel N, Biener D, Kalhs P, et al. Long-term outcome and quality of life of patients who are alive and in complete remission more than two years after allogeneic and syngeneic stem cell transplantation. *Bone Marrow Transplant*. 2002;30(9):619. doi:10.1038/sj.bmt.1703677

Zacher J, Gursche A. "Hip" pain. *Best Pract Res Clin Rheumatol*. 2003;17(1):71–85. doi:10.1016/S1521-6942(02)00108-0

Thyroid Cancer Survivorship Care

Johnny L. Rollins

CLINICAL PEARLS

- Thyroid cancer is the most common endocrine malignancy and is increasing in occurrence. Higher incidence likely is related to the expanding use of diagnostic scans that lead to incidental findings of thyroid cancers.

- Thyroid function tests (TFTs) should be used annually to monitor hormone replacement therapy and arrange for appropriate medication refills. TFTs also should be used 6 to 12 weeks after a dose change to evaluate therapy, when new symptoms arise, and/or in cases involving sudden weight changes of 10 to 15 lb.

- When thyroid cancer is diagnosed before age 40, patients are at elevated risk for low bone mass; monitor calcium and vitamin D levels accordingly.

THYROID CANCER EPIDEMIOLOGY AND SURVIVORSHIP CARE

- General background:
  - Thyroid nodules are common, but fewer than 15% are malignant.
  - Thyroid cancer is the most common endocrine malignancy and is increasing in occurrence.
    - Higher incidence likely is related to the expanding use of diagnostic scans that lead to incidental findings of thyroid cancers.
  - Thyroid cancer rates peak during the fourth decade for women and the sixth decade for men:
    - About 2% of thyroid cancers occur in children and teens.
  - Females have a higher incident rate:
    - Three of four patients with thyroid cancer are female.
    - The thyroid was the fifth leading cancer site for women in 2017, according to the American Cancer Society.

- The World Health Organization classification system identifies four major groups of thyroid cancer:
  - Papillary thyroid carcinoma (PTC)
  - Follicular thyroid carcinoma (FTC)
  - Medullary thyroid carcinoma (MTC)
  - Anaplastic thyroid carcinoma (ATC)
- PTC is the most common type and accounts for 80% to 85% of all thyroid cancer cases.
- Survival rates are highest for patients younger than age of 45 who have PTC.
- ATC is less common (<2% of cases) and is associated with the highest mortality rates (<10% survival at 5 years).
- There does not seem to be an ethnic link, but several inherited genes and medical conditions are linked to thyroid cancer:
  - Multiple endocrine neoplasia (MEN) type 2:
    - — MEN2A and MEN2B
    - — Familial medullary thyroid carcinoma (FMTC)
  - Familial adenomatous polyposis
  - Cowden disease
  - Carney complex, type I
- Risk factors include a diet low in iodine and exposure to radiation:
  - Most common thyroid cancers seen in survivors:
    - — Differentiated thyroid cancers (DTC) arise from the follicular thyroid cells (PTC and FTC):
      - a. PTC: 80% to 85% of all thyroid cancer cases
      - b. FTC: 5% to 10% of all thyroid cancer cases
    - — Survival:
      - a. Excellent prognosis, with a 10-year survival rate around 95%
  - MTC:
    - — About 2% to 5% of all thyroid cancer cases
    - — About 20% to 30% of all MTCs are autosomal dominant (involving inherited genes):
      - a. MEN2A, MEN2B, and FMTC
    - — Peak incidence is at around age 35; peak age for sporadic MTC is 40 to 60 years
    - — Survival:
      - a. 5-year survival 86%
      - b. With older age at diagnoses, advanced stage, metastatic lymph nodes, and/or *RET* mutation are associated with poorer prognoses
  - Thyroid cancer staging:
    - — Refer to the American Joint Committee on Cancer's Staging Systems for Differentiated and Anaplastic Thyroid Cancer (8th Edition) and Medullary Thyroid Cancer (8th Edition) for the most up-to-date tumor staging information

o Clinical tools for transitioning to survivorship:
   — Eligibility criteria for transition of patients with thyroid cancer to survivorship (refer to Figure 16.1)

DISEASE SURVEILLANCE

- Medical history and physical examination (Figure 16.1):

  ■ Detailed focused history: medication-related questions:
    o Any changes in thyroid hormone medications since your last clinic visit?
    o Has the tablet's size, shape, or color changed?
    o Describe how the medication should be taken and ask about the patient's medication routine:
       — Empty stomach versus with food
       — Taking other medications or supplements that can reduce thyroid hormone absorption, such as multivitamins, calcium or iron supplements, a proton pump inhibitor, or other medications that change gastric acidity?
       — Morning or night?
       — Skip or forget thyroid hormone medications? If so, do they take an extra dose the following day?
    o General constitutional questions:
       — Fatigue, tiredness, weight changes, recent illnesses, and/or hospitalizations?
    o Head and neck questions:
       — Voice changes?
       — Swallowing changes?
       — Pain or stiffness?
       — New masses or tenderness?
    o Vision questions:
       — Excessive tearing/dryness?
       — Vision changes?
    o Cardiovascular questions:
       — Palpitations?
       — Chest pain?
       — Shortness of breath?
    o Skin questions:
       — Excessive dryness?
       — Thinning of hair or eyebrows?
    o Endocrine questions:
       — Heat or cold intolerance?
       — Excessive sweating?
    o Gastrointestinal questions:
       — Changes in bowel function?
       — Stomach pain?
       — Nausea or vomiting?

216

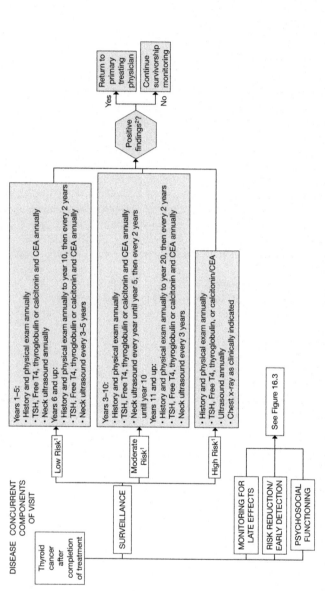

FIGURE 16.1 Thyroid cancer survivorship algorithm (includes papillary, follicular, and medullary carcinoma).

Note: [1] Low Risk: T1 N0 M0, no evidence of disease (thyroglobulin less than or equal to 1 or calcitonin less than or equal to 5; no suspicious lymph nodes or thyroid bed lesions by ultrasound) at 1 year; Moderate Risk: T1 N1 M0, T2-4 N0-1 M0, no evidence of disease (thyroglobulin less than or equal to 1 or calcitonin less than or equal to 5; no suspicious lymph nodes or thyroid bed lesions by ultrasound) at 3 years; High Risk: T2-4 N0-1 M0, stable minimal evidence of disease (thyroglobulin less than or equal to 5 or calcitonin less than or equal to 50; no suspicious lymph nodes or thyroid bed lesions or stable subcentimeter lesions by ultrasound) at 5 years; [2] Positive findings: Enlarging nodules by ultrasound greater than 1 cm, biopsy or confirmed recurrence, rising tumor markers, new evidence of

o Musculoskeletal questions:
  — Hand tremors?
  — Extremity cramping?
o Neurologic questions:
  — Sleeping problems?
  — Problems with concentration or focus?
▪ Focused physical examination:
o Head and neck:
  — Inspection:
    a. Symmetrical smile
    b. Voice
    c. Incisional scar
    d. Swallowing
    e. Oral cavity: moist or dry, teeth and gum problems, ulcers or leukoplakia?
o Palpation:
  — Lymph node assessment (Figure 16.2):
    a. Level I—Submandibular and submental
    b. Level II—Superior spinal accessory and superior jugular
    c. Level III—Midjugular
    d. Level IV—Inferior jugular
    e. Level V—Posterior triangle
    f. Level VI—Pretracheal and paratracheal
    g. Level VII—Intraclavicular and anterior mediastinal (thymic)
o Eyes:
  — Inspection:
    a. Thinning eyebrows
    b. Bulging eyes
    c. Edema
    d. Lid lag
  — Extraocular movements
o Cardiovascular:
  — Palpation:
    a. Pulse rate and rhythm
  — Auscultation:
    a. Heart sounds and rhythm
o Skin
  — Inspection:
    a. Dry, scaly
    b. Increased sweating
o Musculoskeletal:
  — Inspection/observation:
    a. Looking for tremors, outstretched arms with fingers open
    b. Trousseau's sign if the patient has a history of postsurgical hypopara-
       thyroidism

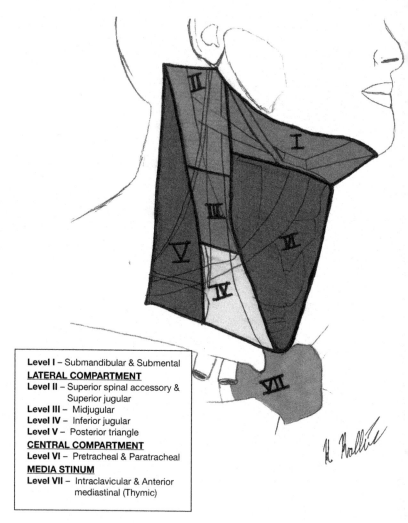

Level I – Submandibular & Submental
LATERAL COMPARTMENT
Level II – Superior spinal accessory &
Superior jugular
Level III – Midjugular
Level IV – Inferior jugular
Level V – Posterior triangle
CENTRAL COMPARTMENT
Level VI – Pretracheal & Paratracheal
MEDIA STINUM
Level VII – Intraclavicular & Anterior
mediastinal (Thymic)

FIGURE 16.2 Head and neck lymph node assessment.

   c. Chvostek's sign if a patient has a history of postsurgical hypopara-
      thyroidism

- Laboratory assessment (refer to Figure 16.1):

   ▪ TFTs should be used annually to monitor hormone replacement therapy and
     arrange for appropriate medication refills. TFTs should also be used 6 to 12 weeks

after a dose change to evaluate therapy, when new symptoms arise, and/or in cases involving sudden weight changes of 10 to 15 lb:
- o Thyroid-stimulating hormone (TSH):
  - — See Table 16.1 for TSH goals
- o Free T4
- o Total T3
  - — Only if taking desiccated thyroid or thyroid extract
- ■ Tumor markers:
  - o Thyroglobulin (Tg) level with antibodies:
    - — For patients with DTC
  - o Calcitonin and carcinoembryonic antigen (CEA):
    - — For patients with MTC

- Diagnostic imaging (refer to Figure 16.1):

  - ■ Neck ultrasound
  - ■ CT scan of chest and neck soft tissue with contrast, if indicated:
    - o Rising tumor markers (Tg or CEA/calcitonin levels) with stable neck ultrasound
    - o History of pulmonary nodules
  - ■ PET or CT:
    - o If this test is needed, the patient likely should be transitioned out of the survivorship clinic

- Monitoring for late effects (refer to Figure 16.3):

  - ■ Refer to Chapter 7 for more information about the most common late effects
  - ■ Salivary dysfunction:
    - o Head and neck referral

TABLE 16.1 Thyroid Hormone Suppression Goals

TSH[a] Goals	Low-Risk Disease T1 N0 M0 NED[b]	Moderate-Risk Disease T1 N1 M0; T2-4 N0-1 M0 NED	High-Risk Disease T2-4 N0-1 M0 Stable Low-Volume Disease
0–5 y since last treatment	Normal <0.5	0.1–0.5	Suppressed <0.1
5–10 y since last treatment	Normal <1.5	Normal <0.5	0.1–0.5
10+ y since last treatment	Normal <2.5	Normal <1.5	Normal <0.5

[a]TSH, thyroid-stimulating hormone, for which the reference range at MD Anderson Cancer Center is 0.27–4.2 mcunit/mL.

[b]NED, no evidence of disease.

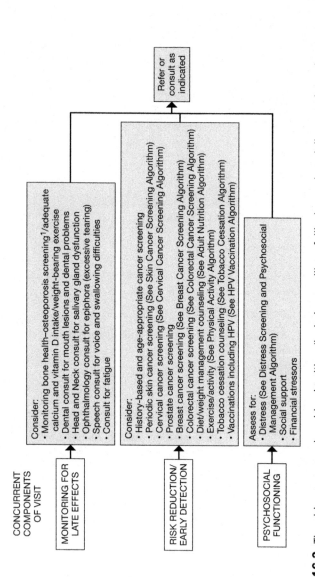

FIGURE 16.3 Thyroid cancer survivorship algorithm (includes papillary, follicular, and medullary carcinoma).

[1]Recommend osteoporosis screening based on the National Osteoporosis Foundation Clinician's Guide 2014 and consider earlier screening as clinically indicated. *Source:* Copyright 2017 The University of Texas MD Anderson Cancer Center.

- Dysphagia:
  - Speech referral
- Fatigue:
  - Fatigue clinic referral
  - Integrative medicine referral
- History of radioactive iodine (RAI) ablation:
  - Dental referral for tooth decay or gum disease
- Thyroid cancer diagnosed before age 40:
  - Monitor calcium and vitamin D levels:
    — Higher risk for low bone mass
    — May need a bone density scan before age 50
  - Patient may need a cardiology referral:
    — Higher risk for hypertension

- Risk reduction and/or early detection (see Figure 16.3):

  - History-based and age-appropriate screening
  - Refer to Chapter 5 for screening and prevention guidelines

- Psychosocial health and functioning (refer to Figure 16.3):

  - Social worker or case manager referral:
    - Financial stressors
    - Social support

- Psychologist or psychiatrist referral (refer to Figure 16.3):

  - Assessment of thought processes:
    - Suicidal tendencies
  - Symptoms of depression or anxiety

CLINICAL EXAMINATION GUIDELINES

- Listen to the patient

- Always ask these questions:

  - How long have you taken your current thyroid hormone dose?
  - Has the pill's size, shape, or color changed recently?
  - Describe when and how you take your thyroid hormone?

- Make sure patients monitor and check their pills:

  - If a pill's color or shape has changed, they should check with their provider to find out if the dose or manufacturer has changed

- If a patient skips or forgets his or her thyroid hormone medication, tell them to take it as soon as they realize the omission or they can take an extra tablet or capsule with the next dose

- Thyroid hormone level testing frequency:
  - Annually if stable; more testing means more adjustments, and a patient can be riding a roller coaster for months
  - At 8 to 12 weeks if the dose is adjusted
  - Immediately in the setting of extreme weight changes (10–15 lb), palpitations, increased anxiety or depressed mood, fatigue or tiredness, or other reasons per clinical judgment
  - Schedule annual follow-ups
- Refer to a reputable radiologist

CLINICAL VIGNETTE

Susan is a 50-year-old woman who had PTC at age 35. Pathology revealed a single focus of a 1.8-cm PTC without extrathyroidal extension with lymphovascular invasion. Microscopic metastases were seen in one of five resected lymph nodes. Susan then received 100 mCi of RAI ablation therapy. She is currently taking Synthroid (levothyroxine [generic]) 137 mcg daily, and her TSH level has been suppressed for 15 years. Her Tg level is undetectable and with negative antibodies per today's labwork. She has relocated and now arrives at your clinic to establish long-term care and follow-up.

Questions

1. Why is younger age at diagnosis important?
   - A. Higher risk for hypertension
   - B. Higher risk for osteoporosis
   - C. Higher risk for heart disease
   - D. None of the above
   - E. All of the above

2. A potential late effect of Susan's treatment that would be extremely concerning is
   - A. Xerostomia/gingivitis
   - B. Low bone mass/osteoporosis
   - C. Palpitations/arterial fibrillation
   - D. Sialadenitis
   - E. All of the above

3. What is an appropriate TSH level goal?
   - A. Suppressed, TSH level undetectable
   - B. Moderate suppression, TSH level 0.01 to 0.27 mIU/L

C. Mild suppression, TSH level 0.1 to 0.5 mIU/L
D. Normal range, TSH level 0.27 to 2.5 mIU/L
E. Normal range, TSH level 2.5 to 4.2 mIU/L

4. Which annual screenings are recommended for this patient?
   A. Breast screening including a mammogram
   B. Cardiology examination
   C. Dental examination
   D. All the above
   E. None of the above

5. Should this patient continue to take the brand-name version of this drug?
   A. Yes
   B. No
   C. Both the brand name and generic versions are acceptable; the patient may take either
   D. Alternate between A and B
   E. None of the above

Answers

1. E
Patients younger than age 40 with a thyroid cancer diagnosis are at higher risk for hypertension, heart disease, and osteoporosis. This most likely is related to old treatment algorithms that recommended suppressing TSH to undetectable levels for longer periods. The current recommendations regarding TSH suppression are not as stringent and allow for adjustments depending upon the TNM staging classification.

2. E
All of these late effects are probable, and the patient has several issues associated with these problems. Xerostomia, sialadenitis, and gingivitis are related to radioactive iodine RAI, which can damage the salivary glands and result in blocked or clogged glands, decreased moisture, dry gums, and tooth decay. Oversuppression of TSH or hyperthyroidism can result in atrial fibrillation and low bone mass that leads to osteoporosis.

3. D
The TSH level should be within defined limits. This patient is at low risk for disease recurrence, and she is 15 years out from disease. Her TSH level should be around midpoint on the reference range. Her thyroid hormone dose can be adjusted up or down depending upon reported symptoms or clinical examination findings. No benefit is associated with suppressing TSH level at this time; suppression will result in worsening or exacerbating side effects and secondary diseases such as hypertension, osteoporosis, and

atrial fibrillation. If thyroglobulin level findings are positive (indicating possible recurrence of disease), the low-normal range is appropriate for a patient if side effects are not an issue.

4. D

All of the screenings listed are important because of this patient's age and number of years on suppressive therapy. Annual breast screening is recommended for all women, as is a cardiology examination when there is high risk for hypertension, atrial fibrillation, and heart disease. A dental exam is needed once or twice yearly for patients who received high or multiple doses of RAI. Susan is at very high risk for tooth decay and gum disease. A bone mineral density (BMD) examination is not recommended annually unless a patient is undergoing treatment for osteoporosis; however, obtain a baseline BMD because this patient had years of suppression therapy.

5. C

For Susan, it is appropriate to change to a generic drug. The advantage is financial savings, but some patients cannot tolerate generic drugs and experience side effects not seen with brand-name drugs. It may be difficult to stabilize the TFT findings because of an absorption complication. Insurance companies now want documentation that supports the need for brand-name medications.

RECOMMENDED READINGS

Camacho PM, Petak SM, Binkley N, et al. American Association of Clinical Endocrinologists and American College of Endocrinology clinical practice guidelines for the diagnosis and treatment of postmenopausal osteoporosis—2016. *Endocr Pract.* 2016;22(Suppl 4):1–42.

Camacho PM, Petak SM, Binkley N, et al. American Association of Clinical Endocrinologists and American College of Endocrinology clinical practice guidelines for the diagnosis and treatment of postmenopausal osteoporosis—2016—Executive summary. *Endocr Pract.* 2016;22(9):1111–1118.

Haugen BR, Alexander EK, Bible KC, et al. 2015 American Thyroid Association Management Guidelines for adult patients with thyroid nodules and differentiated thyroid cancer: the American Thyroid Association guidelines task force on thyroid nodules and differentiated thyroid cancer. *Thyroid.* 2016;26(1):1–133.

Smallridge RC, Ain KB, Asa SL, et al. American Thyroid Association guidelines for management of patients with anaplastic thyroid cancer. *Thyroid.* 2012;22(11):1104–1139.

Wells SA Jr, Asa SL, Dralle H, et al. Revised American Thyroid Association guidelines for the management of medullary thyroid carcinoma: the American Thyroid Association guidelines task force on medullary thyroid carcinoma. *Thyroid.* 2015;25(6):567–610.

Index

complete blood count, 207
comprehensive geriatric assessment
        (CGA), 54
computed tomography (CT) scan
    colorectal cancer, 130
    prostate cancer, 145
    thyroid cancer, 219
concomitant chemotherapy, 28
conditioning regimen, 184
coronary artery disease (CAD),
        26–27
Cowden syndrome, 45
cranial neuropathy, 160
CT scan. *See* computed tomography scan

DCIS. *See* ductal carcinoma in situ
de Quervain's tenosynovitis, 70
*Delivering High-Quality Cancer Care:
        Charting a New Course for a
        System in Crisis,* 4
dental decay, 160
dermatomyositis myositis, 71
diabetes, 173, 175
diet recommendations
    for breast cancer, 119
    calcium supplements, 69
    childhood cancer survivors, 103
    colorectal cancer patients, 132, 137
    low iodine, 214
diet/weight management, 119
differentiated thyroid cancers (DTC), 214
diffuse large B-cell lymphoma (DLBCL),
        168, 169
distress
    colorectal cancer, 133, 134, 136
    definition of, 33
    fertility issues, 39
    financial distress, 134
    head and neck cancer, 161
    lymphoma, 176–177
    prostate cancer, 148
DLBCL. *See* diffuse large B-cell
        lymphoma
donor stem cells, 184

donor types, 185
Doppler ultrasound, 199
doxorubicin, 25, 123
DTC. *See* differentiated thyroid cancers
ductal carcinoma in situ (DCIS),
        110
duloxetine, 29
dyspepsia, 28
dysphagia, 160, 161

echocardiogram
    cardiac dysfunction, 25
    cardiovascular late effects, 26
    screening, 102
ED. *See* erectile dysfunction
electroacupuncture, 89
electrocardiogram
    coronary artery disease, 26
    hematopoietic stem cell transplantation,
        199
embryonal cancers, 94
emotional needs
    anger, 37
    anxiety and depression, 37
    fear, 37–38
    grief, 38
    survivor guilt, 38
empowerment through resilience,
        40–41
endocrine sequelae, 101
endocrinopathy, 101, 102
endometrial, lung, and ovarian
        cancers, 75
energy balance, 48–49
enteritis, 28
erectile dysfunction (ED),
        145, 147
exercise/activity
    breast cancer, 75, 119
    colorectal cancer patients, 75, 132
    endometrial, lung, and ovarian cancers,
        75
extracranial carotid stenosis, 27
eye dryness, 159